AF365236

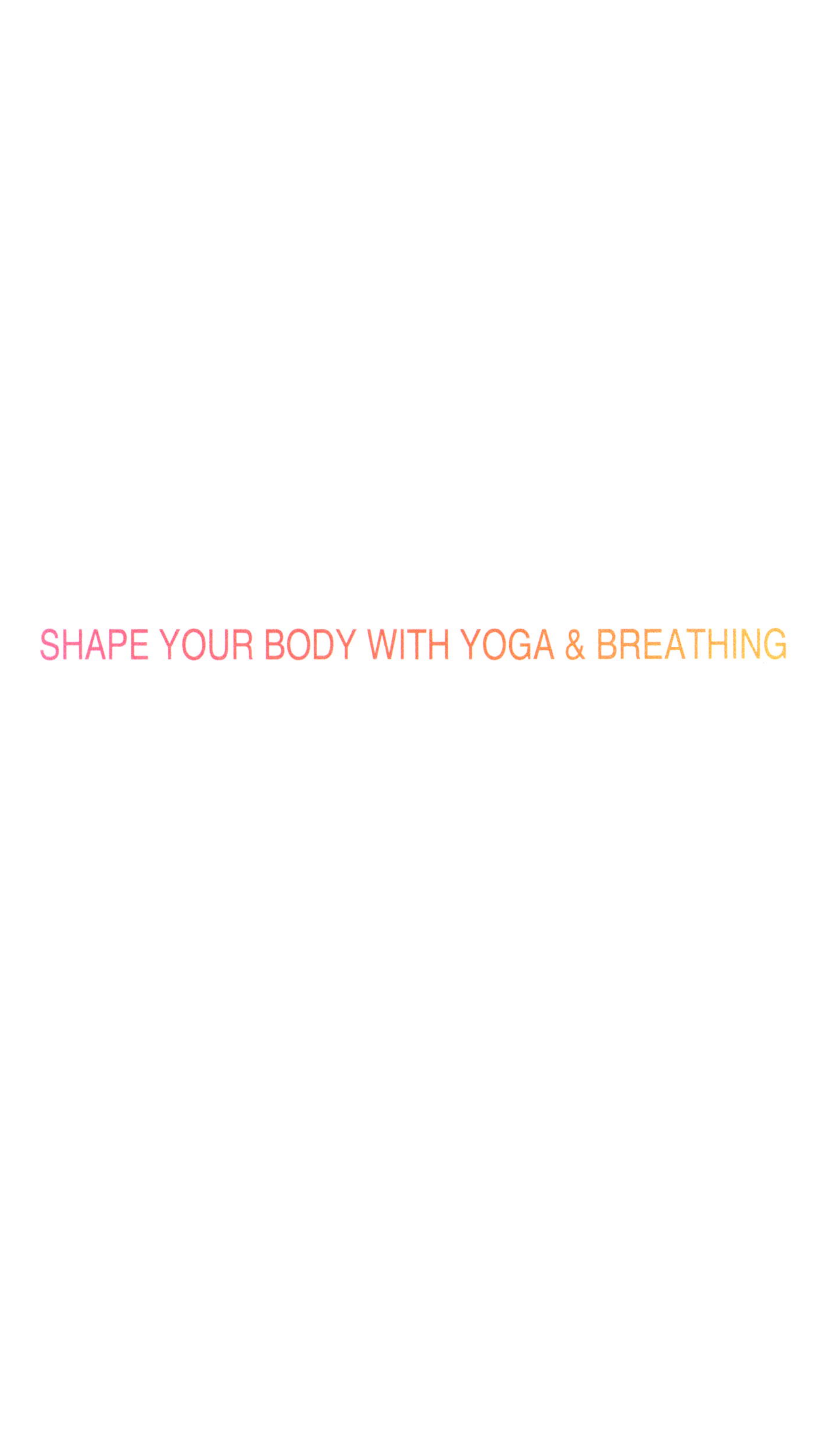

SHAPE YOUR BODY WITH YOGA & BREATHING

SHAPE YOUR BODY WITH YOGA & BREATHING

M.T. Publisher

2015

ISBN I 978-88-91190-40-6

This book is not intended as a substitute for the medical advice of
physicians. The reader should regularly consult a physician in matters
relating to his/her health and particularly with respect to any symptoms that
may require diagnosis or medical attention.

TRANSLATORS: MIKE GUERRIERI & ANNALISA GROVA

Contents

1. PREMISE

"Does Yoga make you lose weight?" During our first meeting my students frequently ask me this question.

In reference to Kundalini Yoga, this question is answered in many kriya proposed by the Master of Kundalini Yoga, Yogi Bhajan; such as those you can find in the manual of Kundalini Yoga "Slim & Trim Yoga Exercises For Women And Meditations". He taught these kriyas to the participants of the Women's Training Course in the summer of 1977.

If you read this text, you would be fascinated by the depth with which Yogi Bhajan talks about being 'overweight'.

> *IF YOU MAKE YOUR BODY*
> *VERY STRONG,*
> *REALLY STRONG,*
> *IT CAN FIGHT OFF ANYTHING."*
> *YOGI BHAJAN*

In other words, as explained by Yogi Bhajan, nervous hunger and compulsive and irrational eating have to do with psychological factors such as stress, discomfort, worry, low levels of energy and a lack of physical and emotional balance. The various kriyas proposed by Yogi Bhajan are useful for stimulating the nervous, glandular, digestive, and circulatory systems; thanks to the stimulation they provide, balance is restored to our body.

This allows us to acquire a calm and deep awareness of ourselves; and due to our heightened understanding of what our body needs, our relationship with food changes. As a result we follow a more healthy and balanced lifestyle.

When speaking broadly about yoga, there have been many studies done on the topic. They confirm that practicing yoga can help with weight loss and prevent the typical weight gain common in middle aged men and women.

I want to point to some interesting research conducted in 2005, published in the journal of "Alternative Therapies in Health and Medicine", referenced by the site: http://www.fhcrc.org.

The researchers at Fred Hutchinson Cancer Research Center, with the collaboration of the National Cancer Institute, analyzed 15,500 healthy men and women of middle age. These men and women were asked to answer a questionnaire about their physical activity between the ages of 45 and 55.
 The purpose of this study was to measure the impact that yoga has on weight, independently from other factors such as diet and other types of physical activity.

 The researchers found that most people gain about a pound a year between the ages of 45 and 55. This is a common pattern as people age but do not adjust their calorific intake in proportion to their declining energy needs.

"However, men and women who were of normal weight at age 45 and regularly practiced yoga gained about 3 fewer pounds during that 10-year period than those who didn't practice yoga," said Alan R. Kristal, Dr.P.H., the study's lead author.

 But the researchers noticed the greatest effect of regular yoga practice was among people who were overweight. "Men and women who were overweight and practiced yoga lost about 5 pounds, while those who did not practice yoga gained about 14 pounds in that 10-year period," said Kristal, a member of the Hutchinson Center's Public Health Sciences Division and a professor of epidemiology at the University of Washington School of Public Health and Community Medicine.

 What accounts for yoga's apparent fat-fighting potential? The researchers suspect that it has more to do with increased body awareness than the physical activity itself.

"During a very vigorous yoga practice you can burn enough calories to lose weight, but most people don't practice that kind of yoga," Kristal says. "From my experience, I think it has to do with the way that yoga makes you more aware of your body. So when you've eaten enough food, you're sensitive to the feeling of being full, and this makes it much easier to stop eating before you've eaten too much."

Study co-author Denise Benitez, owner of Seattle Yoga Arts, agrees. "Most people practice yoga in a way that's not aerobic enough to burn a lot of calories, so it has to be some other reason". The team at the Fred Hutchinson Cancer Research Center now suggests switching to rigorous clinical studies to see if adding yoga to a standard weight-loss program can help people lose more weight or keep it off longer.

2. RIGHT HEMISPHERE: OUR IRRATIONAL PART

"Women who cannot control their eating have no control over their metabolism. It is a problem of the right hemisphere of the brain, it is lack of self-respect, perseverance, affirmation.

"To correct this imbalance take a long and deep breath through the left nostril for 31 minutes a day, for 90 days. Once you can control this you can control everything".

When I read about this meditation, proposed by Yogi Bhajan, I was fascinated. Not only because it was coming from a great teacher, who has the merit of spreading the knowledge of kundalini yoga to the Western world, but also because I needed 'something' that would help me to get out from the labyrinth I found myself trapped in.

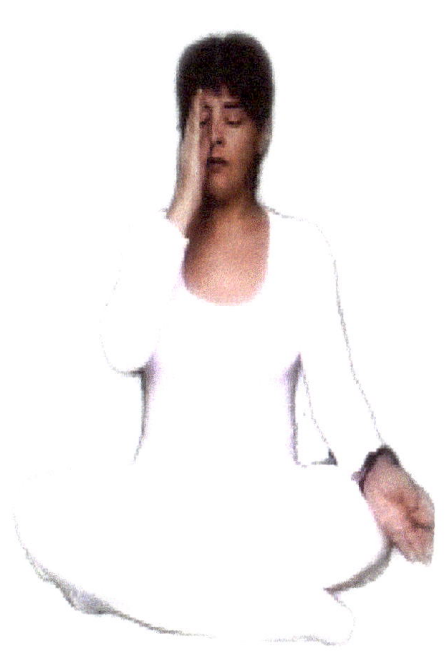

I was facing a period of my life which presented several challenges.

I had some trouble with my family and my job and I had also stopped smoking; because of this I was feeling nervous throughout the day, not getting enough sleep at night and - on top of all of this - dealing with extra weight that I had never had before.

I had tried everything, but I just simply could not get out of the situation I found myself in.

This type of breathing, through the left nostril (described in Chapter 9) was an extraordinary discovery for me, because through it, not only did I become calmer, but I also stopped eating compulsively.

The irrational and compulsive eating has to do with an imbalance of "factors of self-deprivation" in the right hemisphere of the brain.
This can be corrected by activating the left hemisphere of the brain, fighting in this way the impulse of overeating, which originates in the right hemisphere.

At that time I gained even more awareness of the meaning of meditation and of the importance of the emotional part of the brain associated with the right hemisphere.

1. **RIGHT HEMISPHERE -** Irrational and compulsive eating has to do with an imbalance of the factors of self-deprivation in the right hemisphere of the brain. This can be corrected by activating the left hemisphere of the brain, which can then fight the impulse of overeating that originates in the right hemisphere.

2. **DISCOVERIES IN MEDICINE -** The right hemisphere is, in fact, the part of the brain which contains emotions and follows totally irrational rules. Thanks to the progress in the medical and psychological fields, we now know that individuals with bulimia, have higher functionality in the right hemisphere of their brains.

3. **BALANCE BETWEEN RIGHT AND LEFT -** A solution can therefore be found in the balance between the synthetic, concrete, spatial, rational aspect of the left hemisphere, and the intuitive, irrational, emotional right hemisphere. This allows for greater synergy between the two cerebral hemispheres.

4. **PROPER BREATHING -** Few of us are aware that proper breathing can change our relationship to life and can affect our mental and physical wellbeing. Breathing is a purely physical process, so nothing else is needed.

Over time, as you manage to slow down your breathing to a frequency of 3-4 breaths per minute, rather than 13-20 breaths per minute, which is considered normal, you will find enormous benefits.

I want to emphasize the importance of proper breathing. Many of us are actually not breathing properly. We are either doing 'opposite or inverted breathing' or what is known as 'paradoxical breathing'.

In the 'opposite or inverted breathing', while we inhale, our diaphragm rises and during expiration it falls. It's supposed to be the opposite!

In 'paradoxical breathing', the secondary muscles of respiration (scalene, sternocleidomastoid, trapezius, pectoralis minor muscles) replace the functions of the primary ones. In this case, the breath becomes short and superficial.

The use of secondary muscles leads to chronic tension, anxiety, fear, lack of esteem. It is important to understand how the type of breathing we do can affect our lives!

As a yoga teacher I dedicate a lot of time to studying breathing. I'm sure people would overcome many of their problems if they learned how to breathe correctly.

Yet another type of incorrect breathing is what's known as 'collapsed breathing'. That's when we make a short inhalation followed by a very short exhalation (like a puff), that doesn't pull out any air, but makes the abdominals collapse forward.

The areas of the sacrum and lower back also collapse forward, the muscles of the rectum become soft and the rest of the back compensates, bending forward. This type of breathing can lead to depression.

3. OSHO: THE FIRST CHAKRA AND OUR NEED FOR LOVE

The seven chakras are vortexes of energy and vital centers that are found in our body. From the perspective of neurophysiology, the chakras are each associated with one of our organs. When, in each one of us, these chakras are balanced, the energy flows and there is a deep feeling of well being. It is important that these chakras are balanced in each one of us.

This allows the flow of energy within us and creates a deep feeling of well being.

In eating disorders the first Chakra, Muladhara (Root), corresponding to the large intestine, rectum and adrenal glands, is constipated. The yoga postures associated with the first chakra (described in chapters 38, 39, 40, 41, 42, 43, 44), are useful for the flow of the blocked energies in this chakra, freeing yourself from tension and making you more confident.

From an energetic perspective, people who have bulimia and anorexia, for example, have tension in the First Chakra. This is also the Chakra which concerns the relationship with our mother. Since they don't feel accepted, they don't accept themselves. They try to remove fear and feed the emotional voids, thus they eat compulsively.

In this sense, breathing, meditation and yoga postures help to acquire awareness and to become calmer, leading to the release of remote tensions, and creating a sense of self acceptance.

The exercise related to the First Chakra, will be followed by those of the Fourth Chakra (in chapters 45, 46, 47, 48, 49). The Fourth Chakra, Anahata, is also called chakra of love because this chakra is conditioning our ability to receive and to give love. When the Heart Chakra is working properly, we have satisfying relationships; we love ourselves and others and we have no difficulty in feeling accepted. On the contrary, when the Heart Chakra is unbalanced, there is a feeling of not being loved and we have difficulties loving unconditionally (giving love without expecting anything in return) and accepting ourselves just the way we are.

The connection in between Chakras and emotions is well explained by Osho in 'Food and Chakra', from The Divine Melody # 6:

"**The first chakra is concerned with food and the fourth chakra is concerned with love. Love and food are deeply related, joined together. Hence it happens that whenever somebody loves you, you don't eat much. If a woman is loved she remains lean, thin and beautiful. If she is not loved she starts becoming fat, ugly, goes on accumulating; she starts eating too much. Or, vice versa too: if a woman does not want to be loved, she starts eating too much. That becomes a protection -- then nobody will be attracted towards her.**

Have you watched it? If a beloved comes to your home, a friend has come, and you are so happy, and so full of love -- that day, appetite disappears. You don't feel like eating – as if something more subtle than food has fulfilled you, something more subtle than food is inside you and the emptiness is not there. You are full, you feel full.

Miserable people eat too much, happy people don't eat too much. The more happy a person, the less he is addicted to food -- because he has a higher food available: love. Love is food on a higher plane. If food is food for the body, love is food for the spirit.

Now even scientists are suspecting it. When a child is born, the mother can give just milk, bodily food. She may not give love -- then the child will suffer; his body will grow but his spirit will suffer. Just bodily nourishment is not enough: spiritual nourishment is needed. If a mother only gives food and not love then she is not a mother, she is only a nurse. And the child will suffer for his whole life -- something will remain stuck, ungrown, retarded. The child needs food, the child needs love: love is needed even more than food. Have you watched it? If a child is given love he does not bother about food much. If the mother loves the child she is always worried that the child is not drinking as much milk as he should. But if the mother is nonloving then the child drinks too much milk. In fact it is difficult to take him away from the breast because the child becomes afraid: love is not there, he has to depend only on physical food -- the subtle food is missing.

And this goes on happening in your whole life. Whenever you feel that you are missing love, you go on stuffing your body with food -- it becomes a substitute.

Whenever people feel empty and they don't have that thrill that love brings, that zest that love brings, that energy that love releases, they start stuffing their body with food. They have fallen back to their childhood; they are in a regressed state. Children who are given enough love are never addicted much to food. Their spirit is so full: the higher is available -- who bothers about the lower?".

4. EMOTIONAL HUNGER AND BREATHING

It's not uncommon that anxiety, nervousness, stress or our need for love, creates gaps within us that need to be filled.

These needs can also sometimes translate into what we know as emotional hunger. It's an instinctive and irrational hunger; our body is not actually physically hungry; the hunger is not real.

There are various techniques that can help us not give into this emotional hunger.

Aside from the exercise where we breathe through the left nostril, we will also do a meditation to overcome addictions and neuroses.

We will also do some simple exercises of inhalation and exhalation, which will help us to fight emotional and nervous hunger.

This will develop our awareness, giving us an immediate sense of wellbeing and peace, which is needed to overcome stress. Stress can frequently be the source of the urge that can cause us to gulp down food.

By learning the proper techniques for breathing and air distribution, we can gain self-control over food and over our anxiety.

We can then help ourselves not jump irrationally into food.

Of course how we breathe is fundamental.

During the breathing you can mentally repeat a mantra. Mantras are truly effective. The important thing is that you feel comfortable with whatever you choose to repeat. Very often a mantra can be a phrase, a prayer, a thought, a name you love. I often repeat the sound "SA TA NA MA" (which means Infinity, Life, Death, Rebirth), synchronizing the syllables with the inhalation and exhalation.

☑ **SIT DOWN IN A COMFORTABLE POSITION.** Do your best to minimize the noise around you. One good option is to do yoga outdoors.

☑ **START WITH THIS TYPE OF BREATHING** 4/8 (Inhale for 4 seconds and then exhale for 8 seconds). This type of breathing is greatly beneficial in reducing compulsive hunger; it creates feelings of relaxation, patience, and helps with abandonment of harmful habits and old recriminations.

☑ **INHALE FROM YOUR NOSE FOR 4 SECONDS.** 75% of all the work should be done by the diaphragm. When you breathe in, the diaphragm should drop, stretching the lungs, making them dilate, and thus facilitate the access of air.

☑ **EXHALE FROM YOUR NOSE FOR 8 SECONDS.** Very slowly. The diaphragm should rise during exhalation. This will cause the lungs to compress and will facilitate the complete expulsion of air. Continue breathing in this way for 11 minutes. You will experience a state of calmness As you're doing this, focus on the rhythm of your breathing and let any thoughts you may have just slip away from your mind. Do not control them, just let them slip and go away. By maintaining physical stillness you will initiate the meditative state faster.

Proper breathing leads to an inner balance which is essential for taking control over our emotional hunger.

The phase that seems the most difficult is breaking old daily patterns and adding in new ones. Breathing is extremely helpful with that. It helps us move from the old to the new with ease and without constraints. At one point, you will probably actually feel the need to break old patterns. You will feel that your body and mind are asking you for interior cleansing, renewal and transformation.

You will acquire greater awareness and you will begin to feel free and more vital. This is because in that moment you will find yourself being able to control your mind rather than being enslaved by it. You can soar and live a full and happy life, making that moment infinite.

All that's needed is practicing the breathing every day. Just a few minutes a day and before you know it it will become an enjoyable habit.

The yoga exercises described in this book are effective not only because they exercise the body, but also because they renew the mind.

5. INTRODUCTION TO THE EXERCISES FOR THE COLON

For the colon we will be doing some exercises of reflexology, taught by Yogi Bhajan, and also exercises that massage and promote the cleansing and detoxification of the colon (chapters 27, 28, 29, 30, 31, 32, 33, 34, 35, 36).

We know that the colon is the part of the intestine which helps us eliminate waste material from our bodies; the colon and the rectum are both part of the large intestine.

The main function of the colon is to absorb water and parts of our food which cannot be fully digested and take them to the rectum in the form of feces. The colon can be compared to a pipe carrying water.

If there is an accumulation of waste, the pipe becomes clogged and water cannot flow through it.

When a colon is functioning and is cleansed properly this helps prevent problems such as constipation, irritable bowel syndrome, stomach pain, swelling, chronic weakness, acid reflux, skin problems and many other diseases.

It also promotes greater energy intake and a flatter stomach.

The exercises that we will perform, reactivate slow metabolism, increase the secretion of gastric juices and of digestive enzymes, and increase the body's capacity to eliminate. Also they stimulate the meridian points of the stomach and intestines.

6. OVERCOMING FEARS AND NEUROSES WITH MEDITATION

Don't let your mind tell your body that it can't do it. Control your mind, don't let it control you. This is the meaning of yoga and the exercises and meditations described in this book. Once you can control your mind, you can control everything, even emotional hunger.

You will discover that you can do things which your mind thinks are impossible.

The kriya and breathing exercises will prepare your body for meditation, which is nothing more than an access code to reach that higher consciousness we need.

If the mind is not trained, when we're bored, angry, distracted or tired, then we're allowing the thought of food to come and fill the void.

Meditation to overcome fears and neuroses, explained in the next pages, trains your mind to effectively help you in removing any kind of addiction, whether physical or mental.

7. RECOMMENDATIONS FOR PRACTICING YOGA

1	
Do not force your body. Your movements should be natural. Through yoga you will improve gradually. The most important thing to do is to practice consistently.	Three times a week is sufficient. Always warm up your body before starting the exercises.
2	
Find a time and dedicate it to yourself. You can do a 20 to 40 minute program of exercises.	Practice yoga far from meals.
3	
You can do it alone or with your friends, as you wish. Be calm and serene, try to distract yourself as little as possible.	Concentrate on exercises and the rhythm of your breathing.
4	
Even though the place where you do yoga may be small, it should always be clean and well ventilated. The Air is prana, life energy. Do your best to remove anything which may hinder you from the execution of the exercises, for example watches, chains or other jewelry. Wear comfortable clothing and do yoga without shoes.	Keep a clock in front of you. You need it for calculating the time devoted to exercises.
5	
It is important to take care of yourself. It is not just a privilege, it's essential for your health. Whatever the cost, find time to take care of your body and your mind. Practice yoga with perseverance and confidence.	Keep yourself motivated. Continue undeterred, like a warrior fighting for liberation.

8. LONG AND DEEP BREATHING

Sit in a relaxed pose with your hands placed on your knees in gyan mudra (thumb and index finger touching). Alternatively you can sit with your hands relaxed on your lap. For women: put your left hand on top of your right hand while keeping your thumbs touching. For men: put your right hand on top of your left hand while keeping your thumbs touching.

With your eyes gently closed, focus on the root of your nose, the area between your eyes.

Inhale and exhale slowly through your nose in a 1: 1 ratio (breathe in for the same length of time as you breathe out).

The breathing is continuous, there are no stops between the two phases.

Do this without forcing yourself. If you can manage to breathe only 6 times per minute, you will immediately feel a sense of relaxation.

As you inhale your lower abdomen will relax downwards and out; you then continue inhaling into your upper chest.

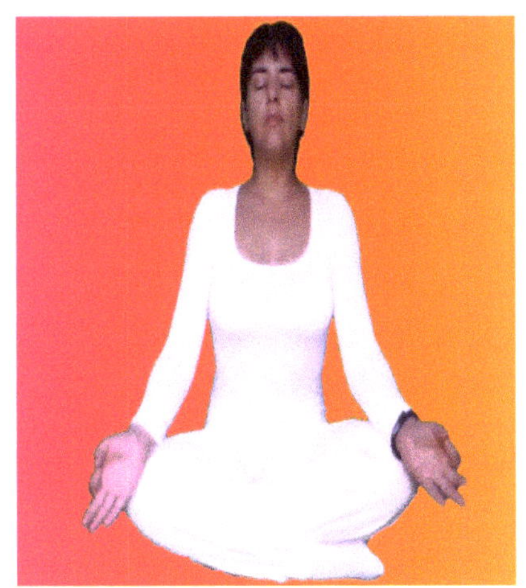

During the exhalation your upper chest lowers and your diaphragm will contract upwards and inwards.

Mantra: The 'Sat Nam' (Sat during the inhalation and Nam during the exhalation), will help you keep your concentration on your breathing as you practice.
Duration: 3-11 minutes.

This breathing, which relaxes, calms, improves clarity of mind, and makes you aware of your thoughts and your surroundings, is the basis of any yogic breathing technique.

It is a technique that will help you to counter emotional and nervous hunger, giving you an immediate sense of well-being and serenity.

9. BREATHING THROUGH THE LEFT NOSTRIL

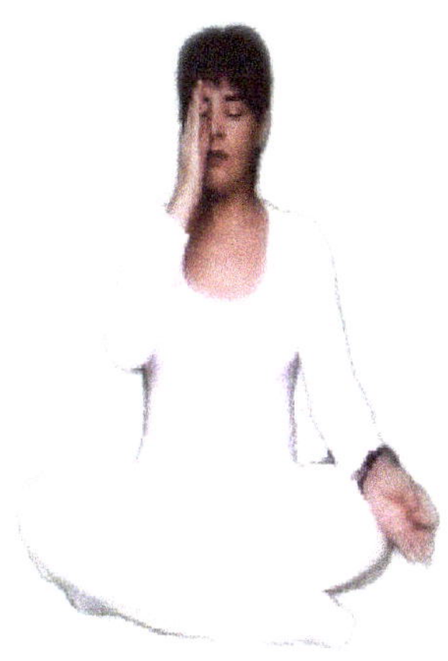

This breathing is done through the left nostril.

Both the inhalation and exhalation occur through the nose in a 4:8 proportion (4 seconds of inhalation followed by 8 seconds exhalation).

You should attempt to do a total of five breaths per minute. The breathing is continuous, there are no apneas or stops between the two phases.

The 'Sat Nam' (Sat during the inhalation and Nam during the exhalation) will help you focus better on your breathing as you practice.

Sit in a relaxed pose.

With your eyes gently closed, focus on the root of your nose. Close your right nostril with your right thumb (the other fingers are relaxed and facing up).
Inhale deeply and exhale, both through the left nostril.

This long, slow and deep breathing, acts on the channel Ida, in other words, the flow of the left nostril, the lunar channel. This type of breathing is useful when you are agitated, upset or angry, and even when the irrational and uncontrolled hunger strikes you.

Over time you will realize how pleasant this type of breathing is and you will build up to doing 31 minutes of it.

Breathing through the left nostril has been recommended many times by Yogi Bhajan:

"Women who cannot control their eating have no control over their metabolism. It is a problem of the right hemisphere of the brain, is lack of self-respect, perseverance, affirmation. To correct this imbalance breathe long and deep through the left nostril for 31 minutes a day for 90 days. This should be a long and deep breathing through the left nostril, without pressure on the diaphragm".

10. 1° EXERCISE: LOSE WEIGHT AND TONE WAIST AND LEGS

This exercise helps you lose weight and tone your waist and legs.

Repeat the movement 10 times, alternating legs.

Always remember to inhale when lifting the leg and exhale when lowering it.

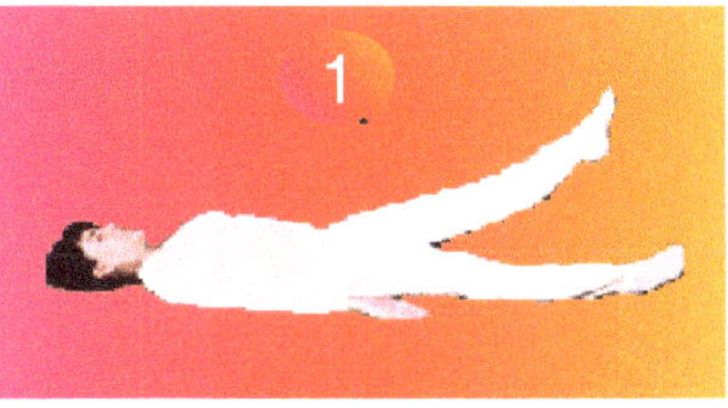

1) Lie on your back, relaxing your arms at your sides. Inhale and raise your left leg 30 cm (12 in). Exhale and lower it.

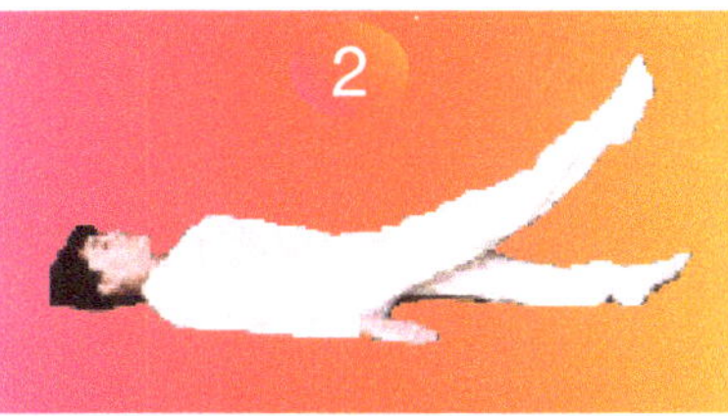
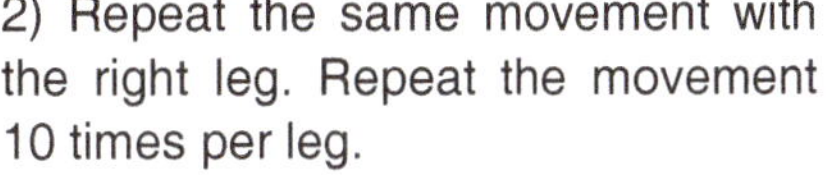

2) Repeat the same movement with the right leg. Repeat the movement 10 times per leg.

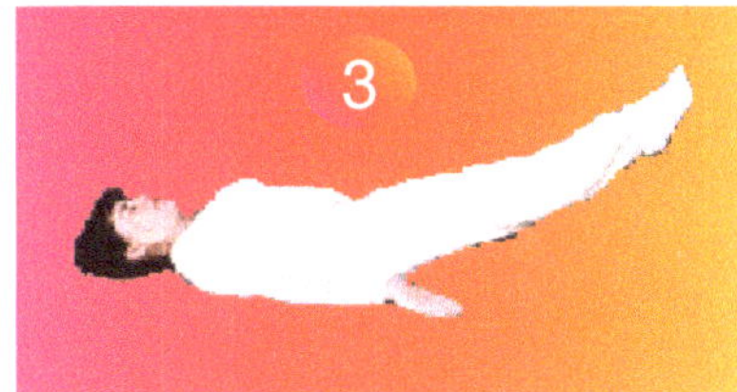

3) At the end of the alternating movements, lift your legs together at 30 cm (12 in) and hold them there for 1 minute, while breathing through your nose slowly and deeply.

11. 2° EXERCISE: LOSE WEIGHT AND TONE WAIST AND LEGS

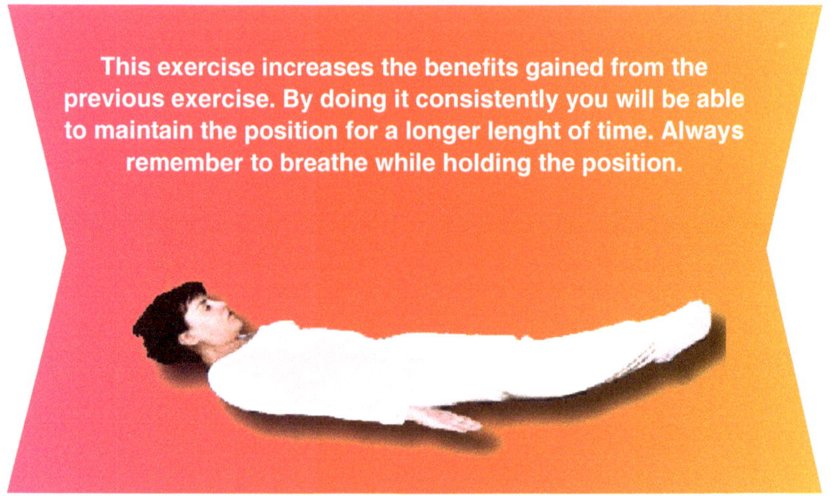

Stay on your back, relaxing your arms at your sides.

Breathing normally, lift your head and legs about 45 cm (about 18 in).

Hold the position for 3 minutes.

When you are tired, relax for 5 minutes. You should still be lying on your back; take slow, deep breaths.

12. 3° EXERCISE: LOSE WEIGHT AND TONE WAIST AND LEGS

1) Lie on your back and inhale deeply.
2) Sit up as you exhale and make sure you're keeping your back straight.

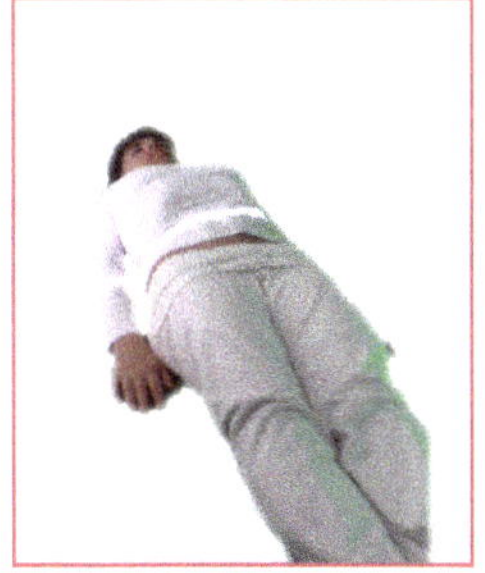

3) As you're continuing to exhale bend forward and grab your toes. If you can't reach your toes, you can grab your ankles or calves. As you inhale, lie down again.

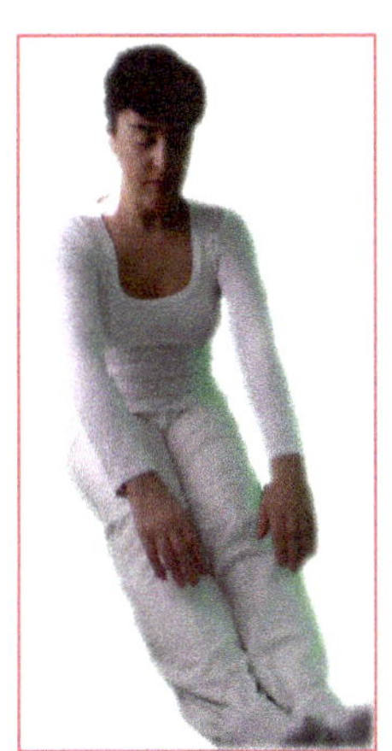

Perform this exercise for 2 minutes.

Try to keep your legs straight, without bending your knees.

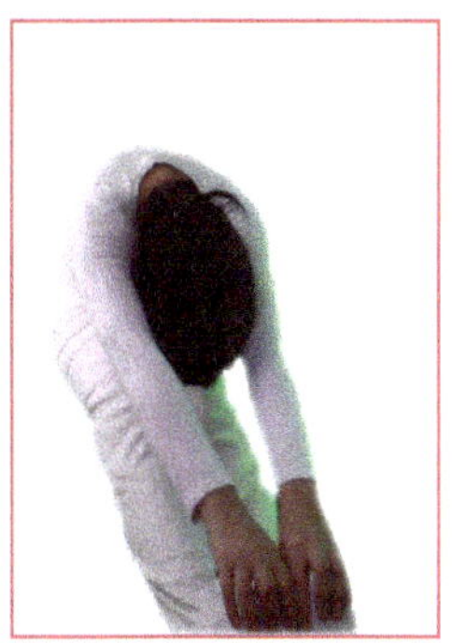

Repeat the 1st, 2nd and this 3rd exercise of this series "Lose weight and tone waist and legs".

Then do the exercise "Breathing through the left nostril", as described in Chapter 9.

13. Series to lose weight and tone your thighs

Do this exercise for 3 minutes with vigorous and rhythmic movements. This exercise will release tension in the back, slimming and toning the thighs. Sit. Spread your legs out as much as possible, keep your torso straight. Inhale while in this position and exhale while bending downward.

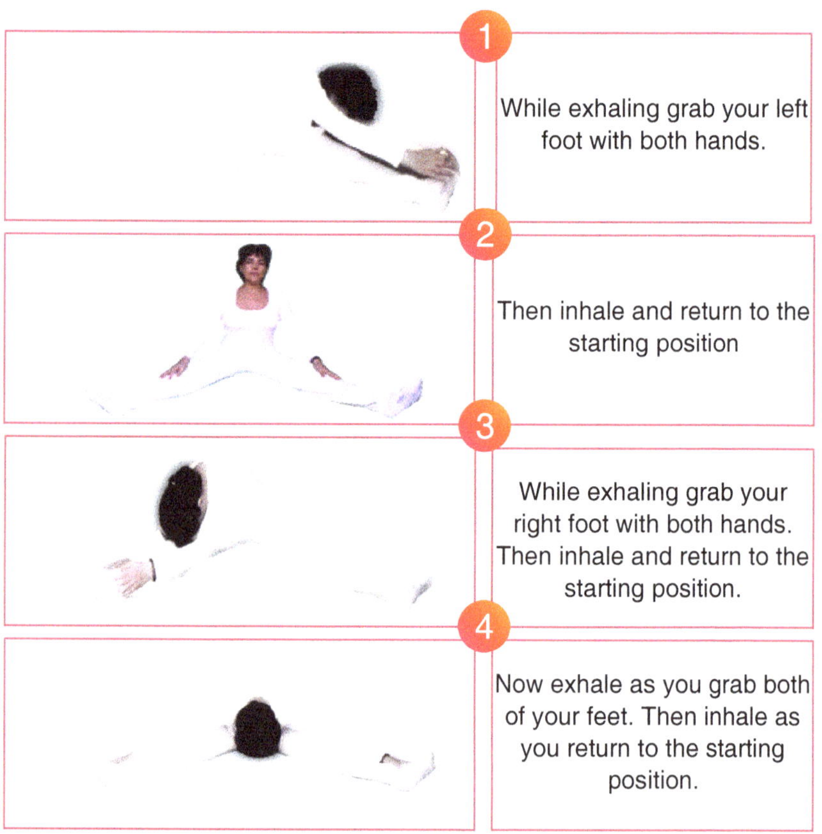

1 While exhaling grab your left foot with both hands.

2 Then inhale and return to the starting position

3 While exhaling grab your right foot with both hands. Then inhale and return to the starting position.

4 Now exhale as you grab both of your feet. Then inhale as you return to the starting position.

Relax on your back for 3 minutes.
Repeat the entire exercise two more times.

14. 1° EXERCISE: SLIMMING BELLY AREA

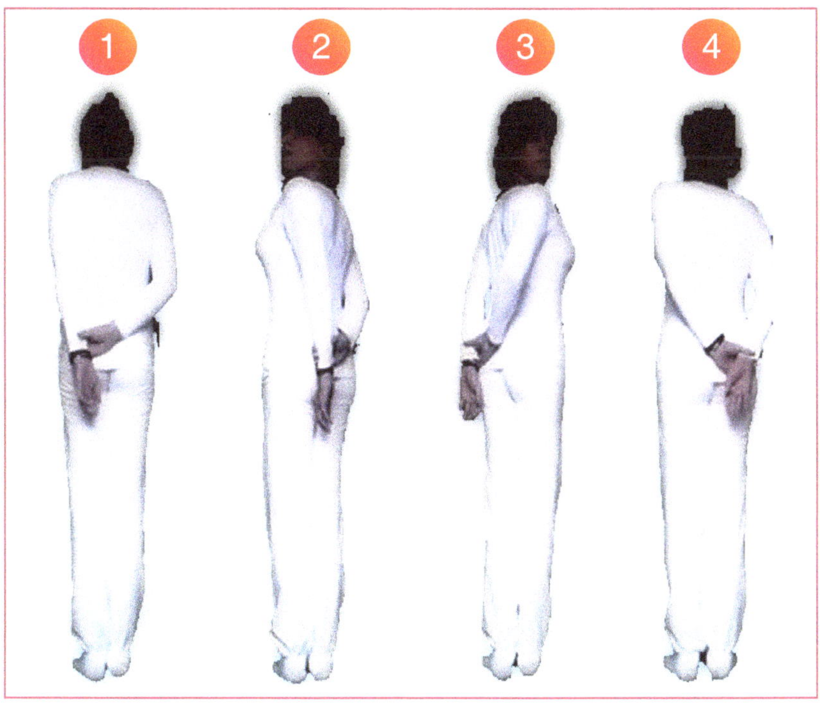

1) While standing, bring the right arm behind your back, grab your left wrist at your waist line.
2) While inhaling twist your torso to the left.
3) Then as you exhale twist your torso to the right. Continue for 1 minute, as you continue to twist your torso to the left and right.
4) Now change hands and twist your torso to the right as you inhale and then to the left as you exhale.
Continue these movements for 1 and a half minutes.

15. 2° EXERCISE: SLIMMING BELLY AREA

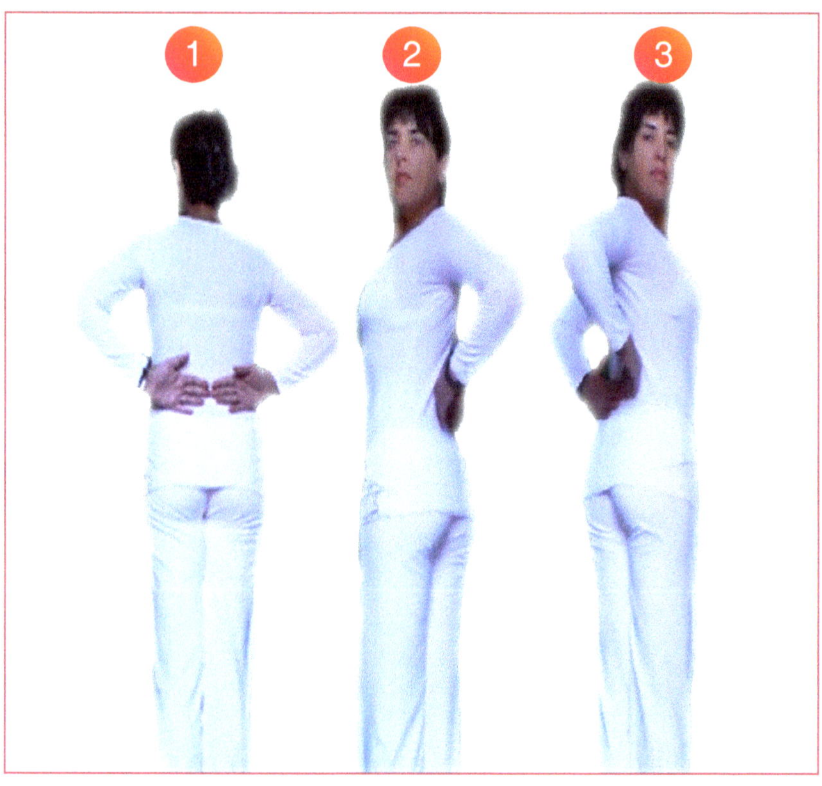

1) While standing, place your hands behind you. The back of your hands should be placed on your lower back.

2) Twist your torso to the left as you inhale.

3) Then twist your torso to the right as you exhale.

Continue this alternating movement for 1-3 minutes.

16. 3° EXERCISE: SLIMMING BELLY AREA

1) Still standing, place your hands behind you. The back of your hands should be placed on your lower back like in the previous exercise. Begin to rotate your whole upper body clockwise as if making wide circles.

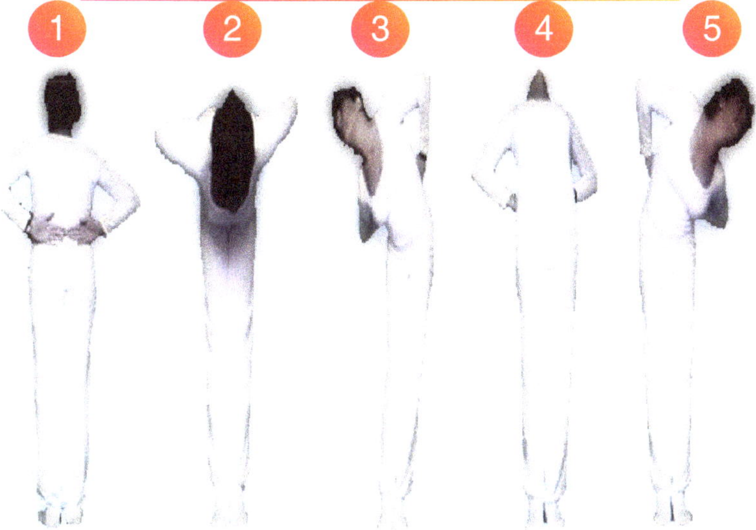

2) Continue by bending forward.

3) Then bend all the way to the right.

4) Then stretch your torso all the way back.

5) And finally bend your torso all the way to the left and then back to the initial forwards bent position.

Continue for 1 minute. Then relax for 3 minutes. Repeat the 1st, 2nd and this 3rd exercise of the series "Lose weight in the stomach / belly area" another time.

17. 1° EXERCISE: LOSE WEIGHT AND TONE YOUR HIPS

This exercise is excellent for the hips and it is beneficial for all the organs in the abdominal area. This entire exercise should be done using the hips, so make sure that you're not using the lower parts of your legs. It is also an exercise that adjusts the hips which then returns the pelvis to the appropriate position. The pain you'll start to feel indicates that the liver has begun working.

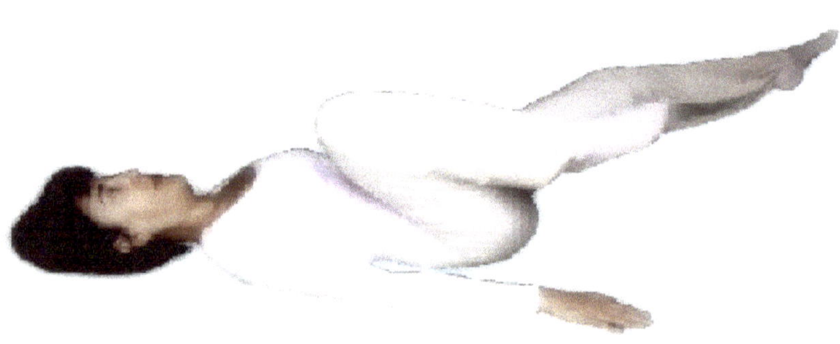

Lie on your back with your arms relaxed at your sides. Breathe normally.

Then bring one of your knees to your chest while moving the other one away.

Continue by alternating knees.

Perform the exercise for 3 minutes.

18. 2° EXERCISE: LOSE WEIGHT AND TONE YOUR HIPS

While lying on your back, spread your legs as much as possible and spread your arms backwards
.
Keep your head on the floor and, using your heels and hands as leverage, inhale as you lift up your pelvis as much as possible.

Then exhale as you return to the starting position.

1

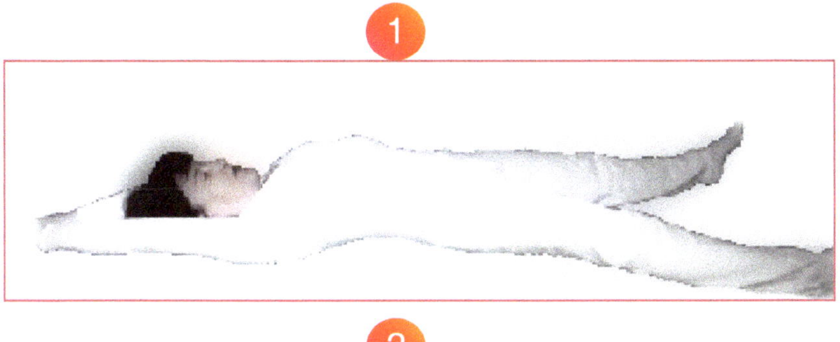

2

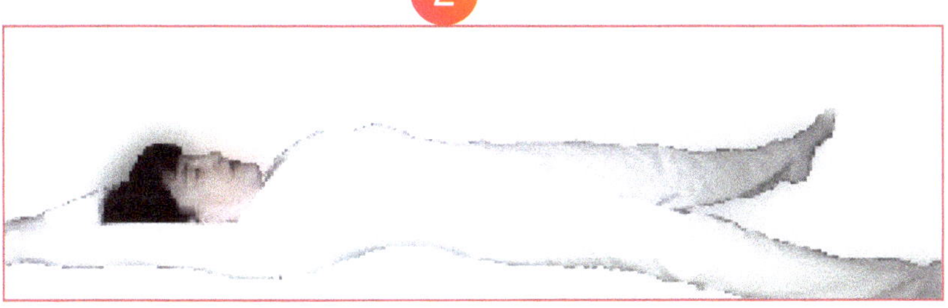

Continue doing this at maximum speed for 1 minute.
Then relax for 1-5 minutes.

19. 3° EXERCISE: LOSE WEIGHT AND TONE YOUR HIPS

Riding the camel will make you sweat and open all your capillaries.

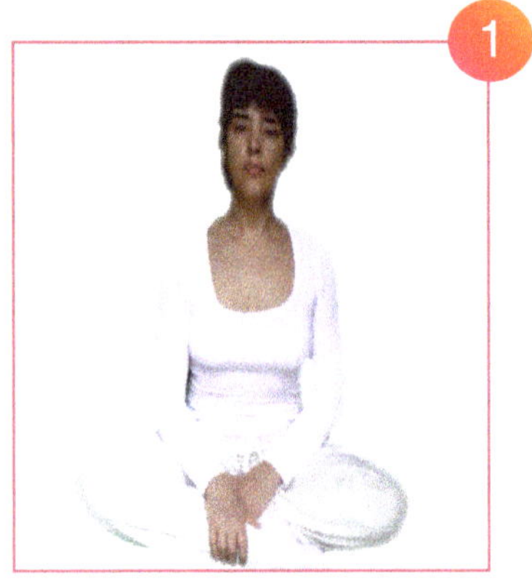

Sit in easy pose, grab your ankles.

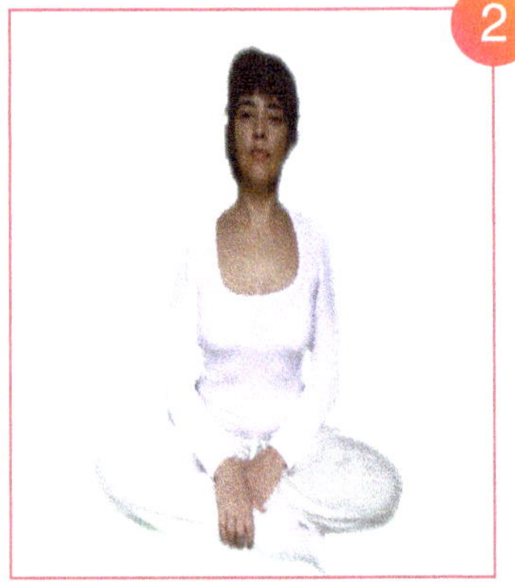

As you inhale, flex your spine forward.

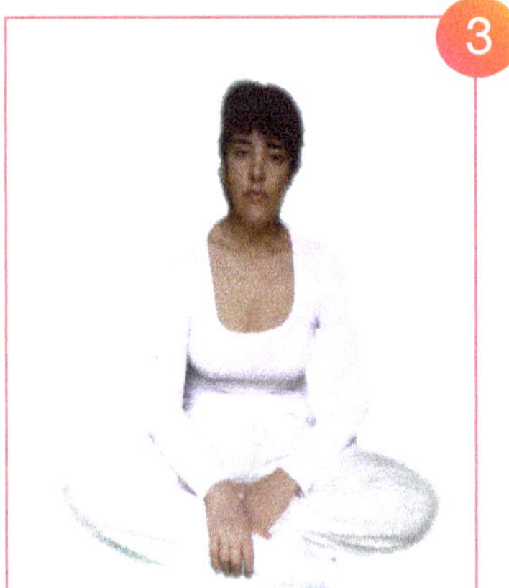

As you exhale flex your spine backward. With your eyes closed tune the movement of the spine with your breath.

Continue for 3 minutes. Then relax on your back as you let your thoughts flow away.

20. 1° EXERCISE: REDUCE HIPS AND BUTTOCKS

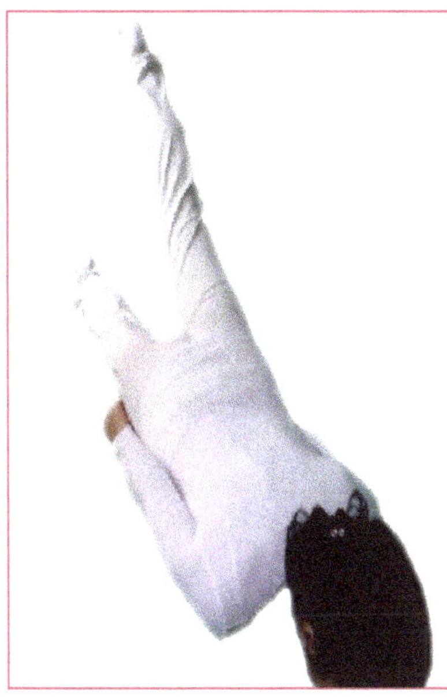

Lie on your stomach, with your chin on the floor.

Your arms at your sides and your hands closed into fists.

As you inhale raise one of your legs as much as possible while still keeping it straight.

Hold the position for a few seconds and then lower it as you exhale.

Then repeat the exercise with the other leg.

Relax for a bit and then perform the exercise two more times while alternating legs.

Then repeat the exercise 3 more times.

Always remember to alternate your legs.

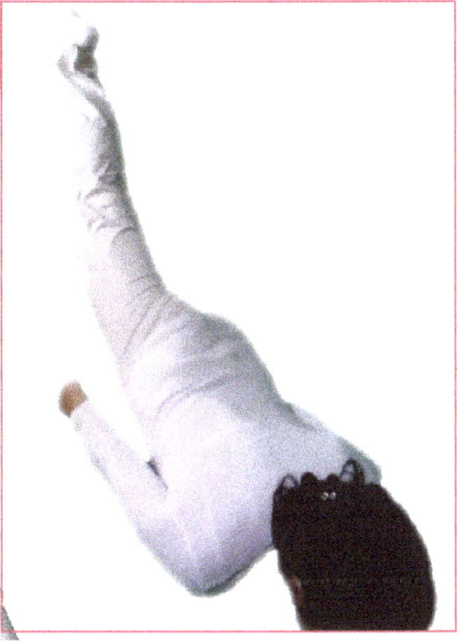

21. 2° EXERCISE: REDUCE HIPS AND BUTTOCKS

Continue this movement for 3 minutes. Then relax.

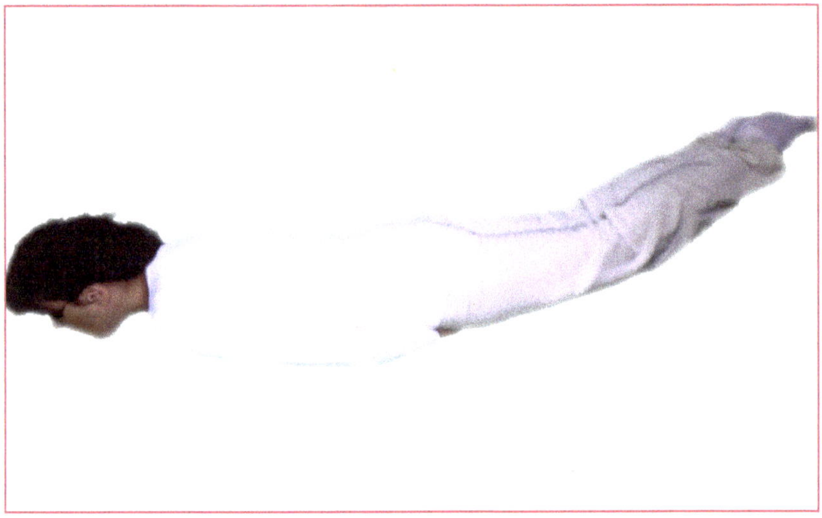

Lie down on your stomach, with your chin on the floor.

Place your arms to your side and your fists should be near your groin area.

As you inhale raise both legs together (at least 20 cm, about 8 in).
Hold them in that straight raised position for a few seconds, and then exhale as you lower them.

22. 3° Exercise: reduce and buttocks

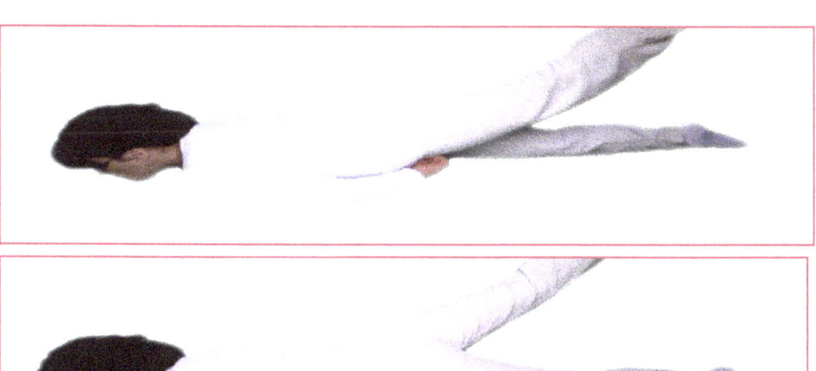

Lift your legs one at a time alternating them up and down. You should be following the breathing pattern described in the previous exercises, synchronizing your movements with a long deep breathing. Continue doing this for 1 and a half minutes.

Then lift both legs and keep them in a straight raised position for 1 and a half minutes. Always accompany the lift with long deep breathing. Relax for 5 minutes. Repeat the exercise and then relax. Repeat the exercise again and relax once again.

23. DIAGONAL STRETCH

This exercise guarantees the maximum relaxation of the spine. Repeat this exercise 4 times per side.

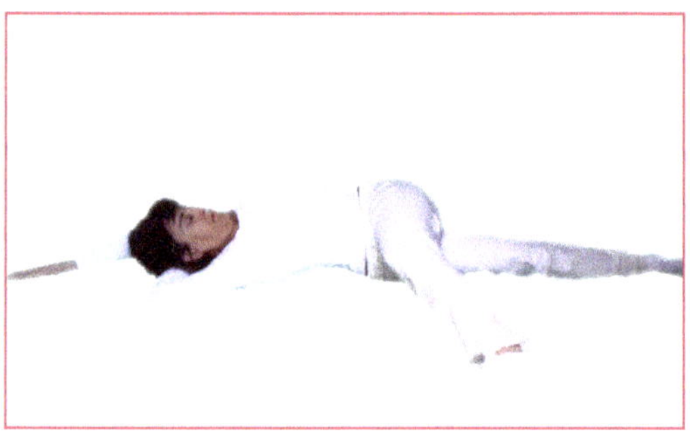

Lie down on your back, put your right hand under your head and bring the left arm backward.

While inhaling through your nose, bring your left leg over your body, and lower it until it touches the ground to your right in a diagonal stretch.

Hold the position for 1 minute, while breathing slowly and deeply. Relax.

Now place your left hand under the head and your right arm backwards.

Slowly bring your right leg above your body, and lower it until it touches the ground to your left in a diagonal stretch.

Hold this position for 1 minute, while breathing slowly and deeply.

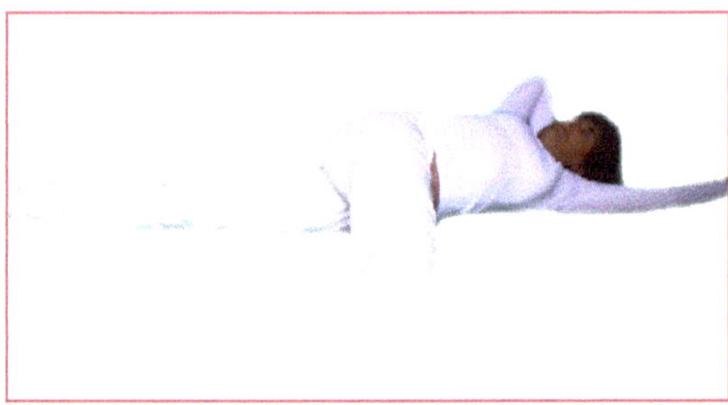

Then change side again. Relax.

24. 1° EXERCISE: SLIM DOWN THE ENTIRE BODY

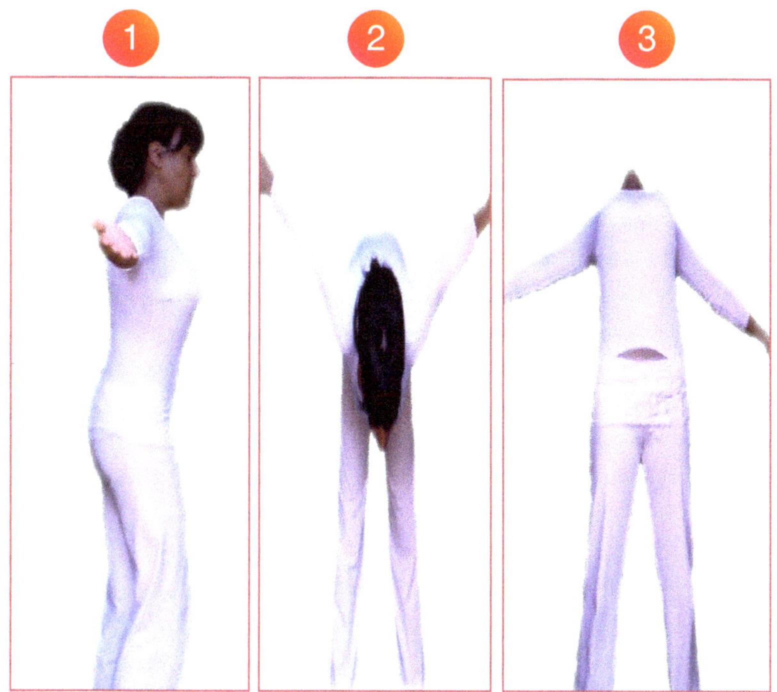

Repeat this exercise for 5 minutes. Then relax for 3 minutes while breathing through your left nostril.

1) Stand with your feet about shoulder-width apart, arms and hands outstretched to your sides and parallel to the ground.

2) Bend your body forward as much as possible. Then return to the starting position.

3) Bend your body backwards.

25. 2° EXERCISE: SLIM DOWN THE ENTIRE BODY

**Repeat this exercise for 5 minutes.
First to the left, then to the right.
Then relax for 3 minutes with long and deep breathing.**

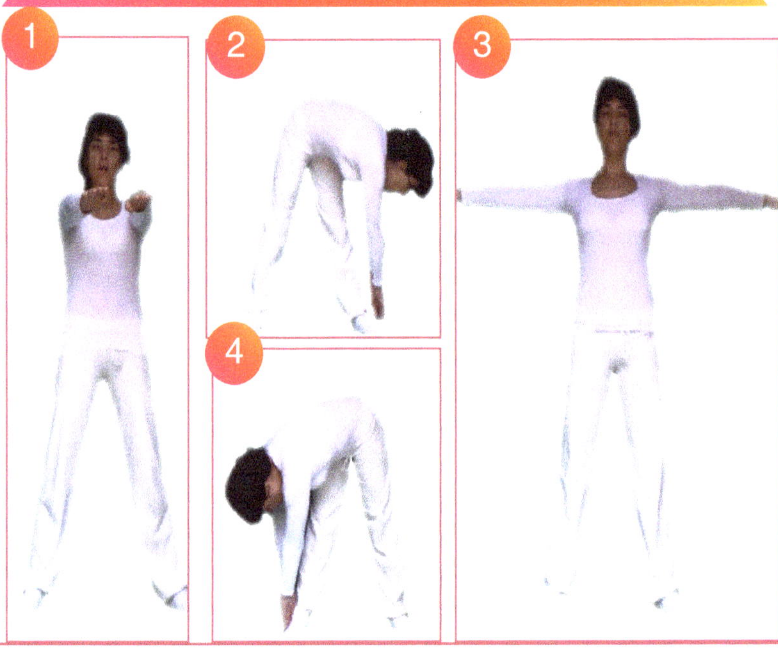

1) Stand with your legs about shoulder-width apart, arms completely stretched forward and parallel to the ground.

2) Twist your torso to the left, and then as you exhale, bend downwards and stretch your arms towards your left foot.

3) As you inhale come back up straight with your arms outstretched to the sides of your body.
4) Repeat the movement to the right side.

26. 3° EXERCISE: SLIM DOWN THE ENTIRE BODY

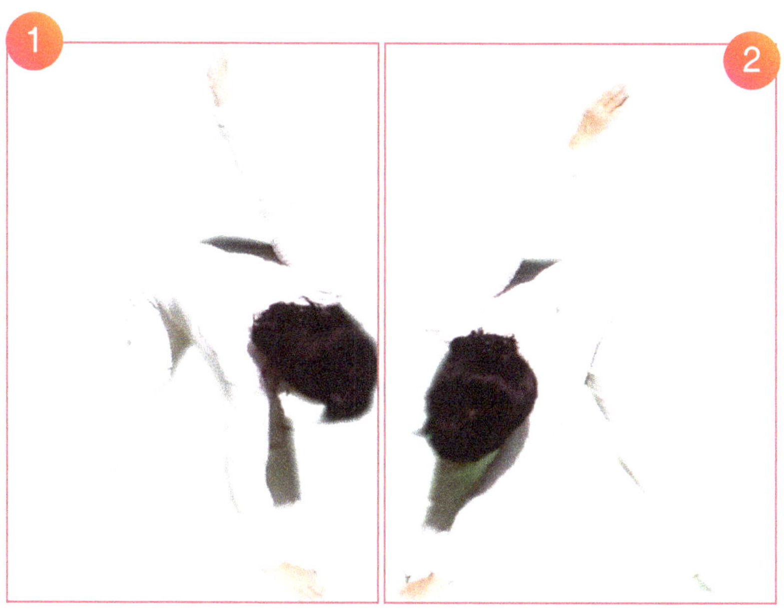

1. While standing, outstretch your arms to the sides of your body, your arms should be parallel to the ground. Bend your torso at the waist, bringing your left hand to your right foot. The right arm is still stretched out above you.
2. Then bend your torso to the left, making the opposite movement with the right hand towards your left foot. These movements should be done one after another; you should not go back to the starting position in between.

Do this exercise for 5 minutes. Alternate movements to the left and to the right while breathing slowly and deeply. Then relax for 3 minutes. Repeat the 1st, 2nd and 3rd exercise of this series: "Slim down the entire body" again. Then relax again for 3 minutes.

27. 1° EXERCISE FOR THE COLON:

TWIST LEFT RIGHT

This exercise is very interesting because it applies pressure on the outside of the feet.

Therefore, this is an exercise that massages, cleanses and detoxifies the colon.

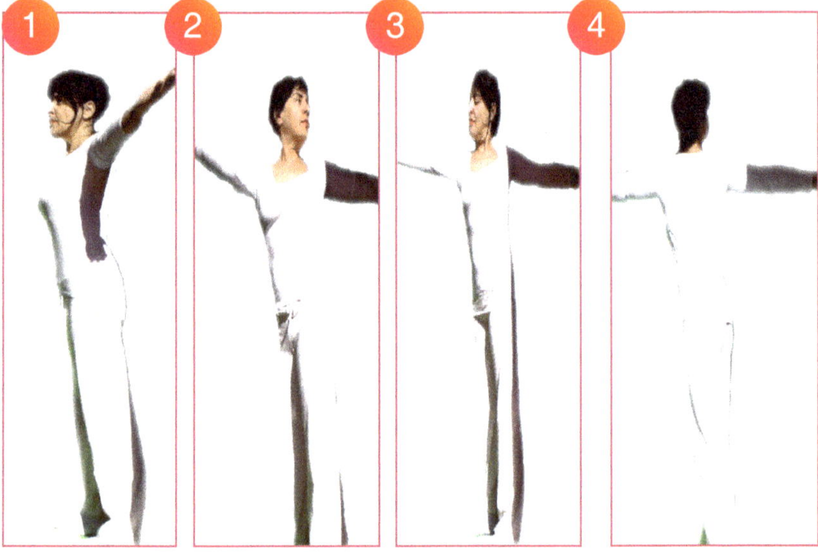

1) Your feet should be shoulder width apart, and your weight should be placed on the outer edges of your feet. Lift your arms to your sides. Your palms should be facing forward at about 45 degrees. Rotate your torso from the waist, 2) to the left, then 3) back to the center, and finally 4) to the right. Each of these movements should be performed at a rate of 3 seconds per cycle. As usual ensure that you're breathing slowly and deeply through your nose.

Total time for this exercise: 3 minutes.

28. 2° EXERCISE FOR THE COLON:

TWIST LEFT RIGHT

Do this exercise for 5 minutes.

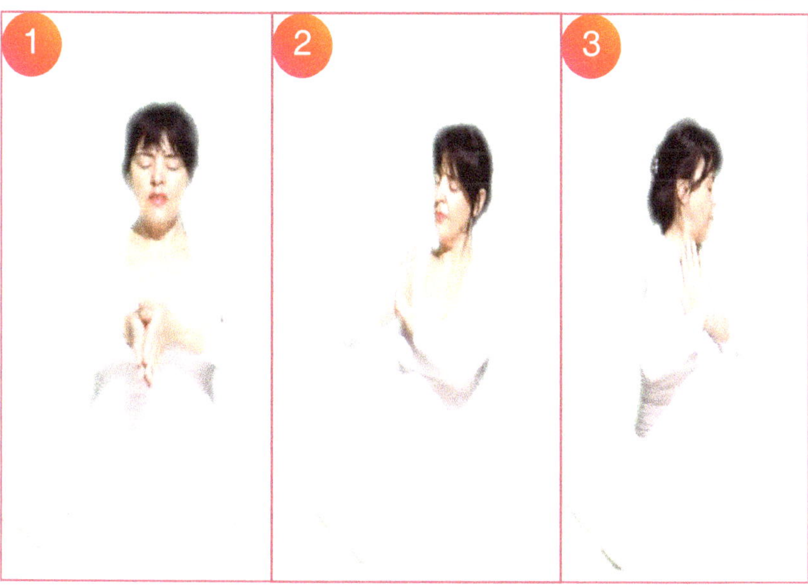

1) Sit in an easy position and bring your hands in front of the right shoulder, in the mudra of prayer, thumbs crossed one over the other.

2) Keep your hands in front of the right shoulder and turn your torso rhythmically to the right.

3) Then turn your torso to the left. As you're doing this, always remember to breathe slowly and deeply through your nose.

29. 3° EXERCISE TO CLEAN THE COLON: ARMS IN A CIRCLE

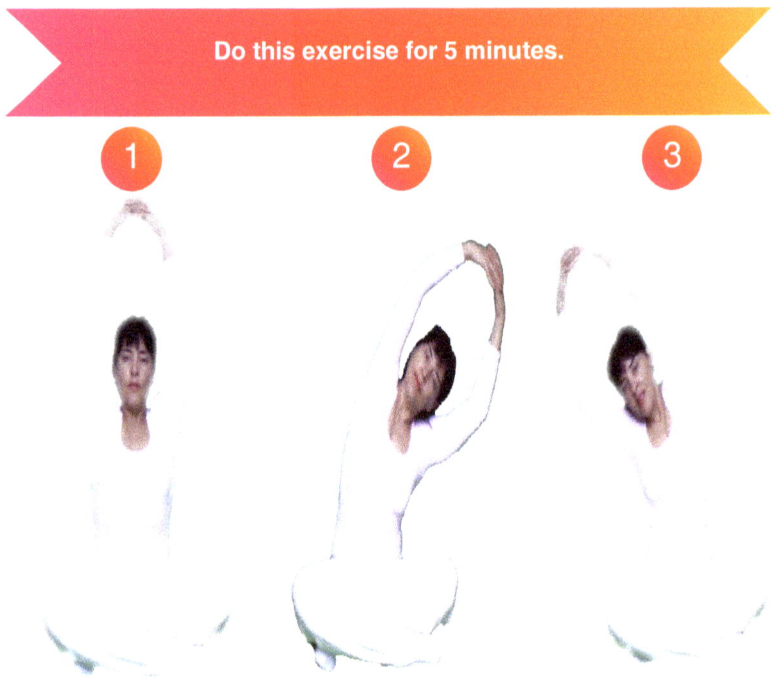

1) Sit in an easy pose, interlock your hands above your head, as if you're forming a circle with your arms.

2) As you inhale, incline your torso as much as possible to the left.

3) Then as you exhale, almost rhythmically, incline your torso to the right.

30. 4° EXERCISE TO CLEAN THE COLON: SHAKING ARMS

Do this exercise for 5 minutes.

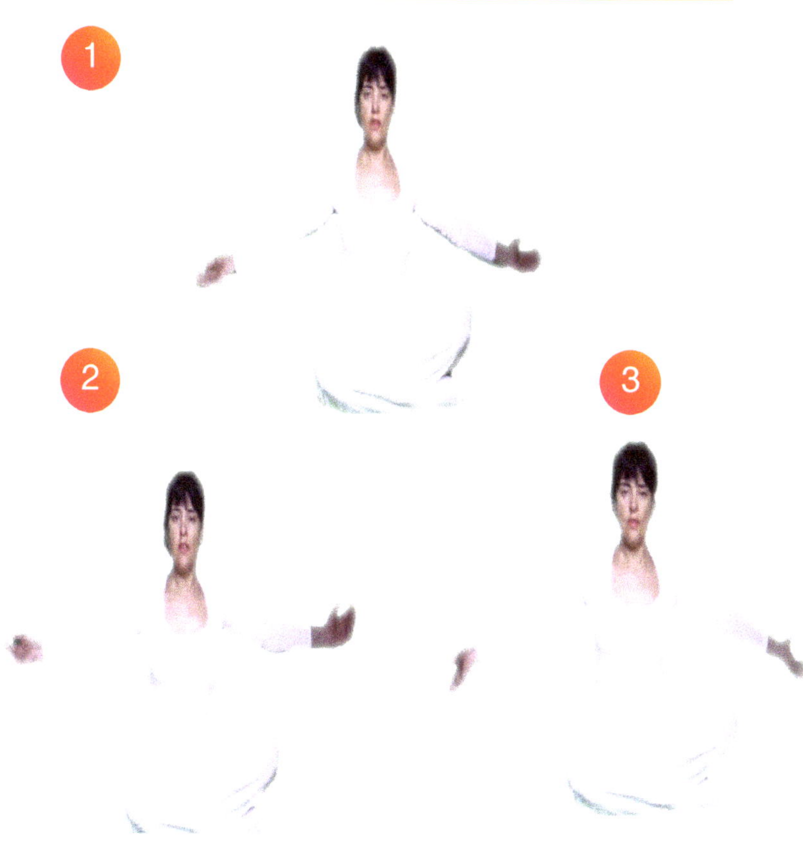

Sit in easy pose. Extend your arms out, forming an angle of 30 degrees down and bring your palms upward.

Keeping your shoulders relaxed and your hands relaxed and heavy, gently shake your arms so that your hands 2) go up and 3) down.

31. 5° EXERCISE TO CLEAN THE COLON: THE PENDULUM

Perform this exercise for 3 minutes.

1) Sit on your heels (Rock Position). Overlap your hands and press them against the abdomen, at the height of your navel.

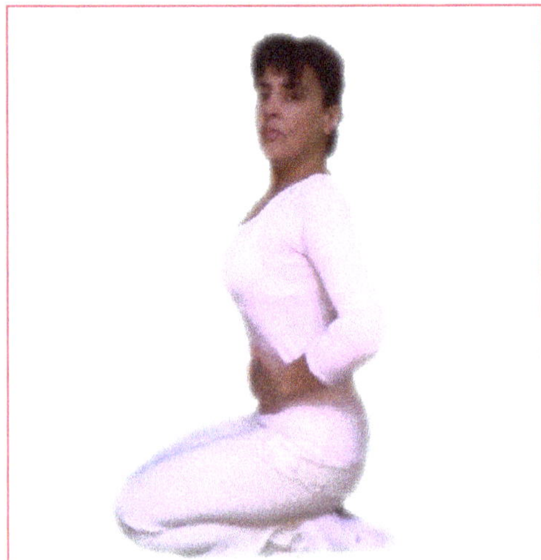

2) Bend your torso forward, bringing your forehead to the ground.

Swing your hips rhythmically from right to left and from left to right like a pendulum.

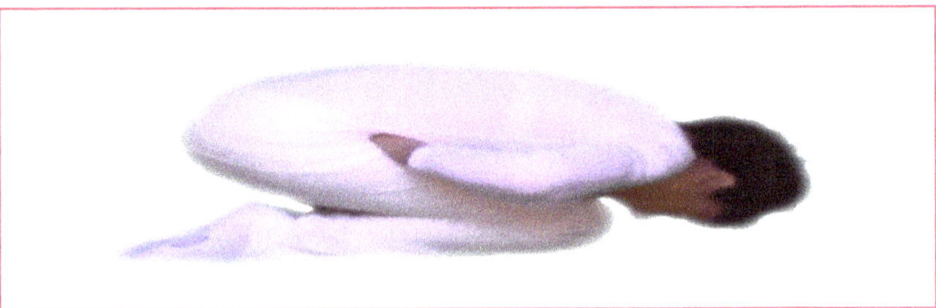

32. 6° EXERCISE FOR THE COLON:

LIFTING FOREARMS

Perform this exercise for 5 minutes.

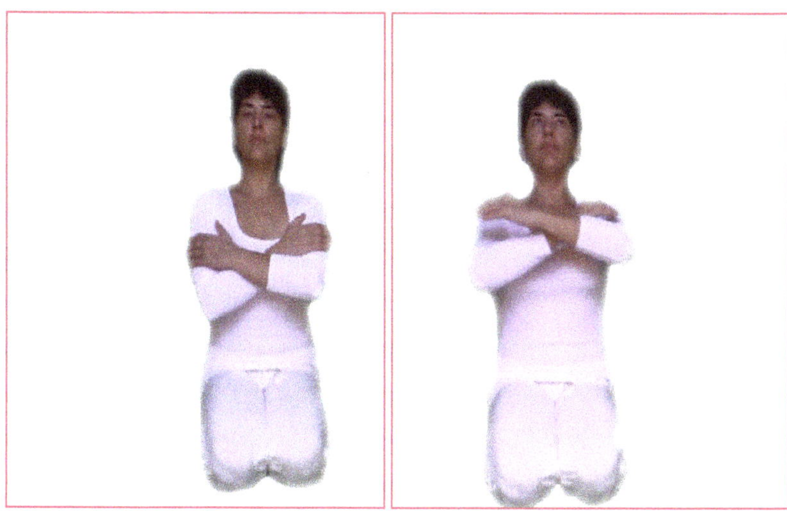

Cross your arms in front of you so that each of your hands is rested on the opposite arm.

Rhythmically raise your forearms quickly and then quickly return to the starting position.

To do this exercise properly you should be striking your arms rather forcefully on the way back down.

33. 7° EXERCISE FOR THE COLON:

SWINGING ARMS

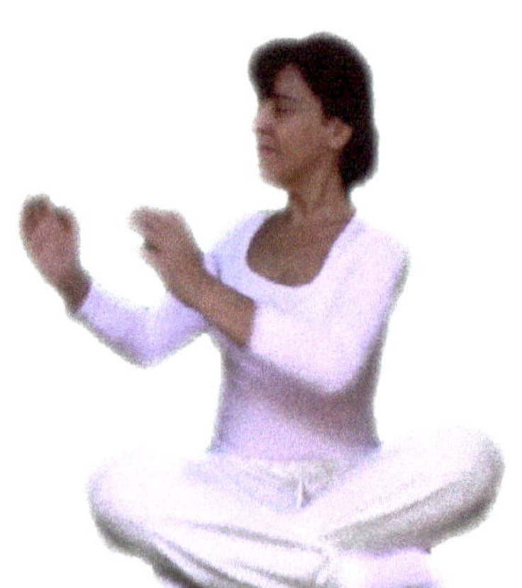

1) Sitting in a comfortable position, inhale as you rhythmically turn your torso to the right, swinging your arms upwards and to the right (hold for 1 second).

Perform this exercise for 1 minute.

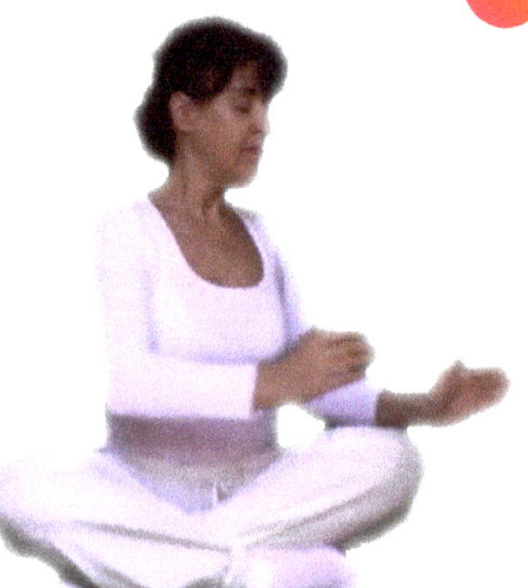

2) Then as you exhale, let your arms swing down and to the left (hold for 1 second).

34. 8° EXERCISE FOR THE COLON: ARMS CROSSED

Do this exercise for 2 minutes.

1) Extend your arms out, parallel to the floor, palms facing upward.

2) With fast and rhythmic movement, raise and cross your arms, then return to the starting position.

Breathe slowly and deeply through your nose during the exercise.

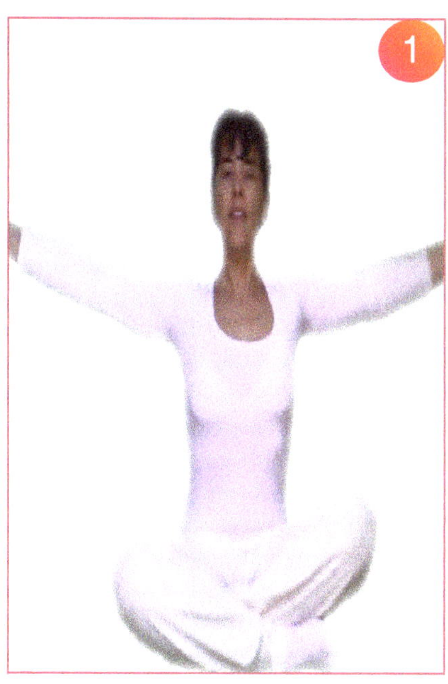
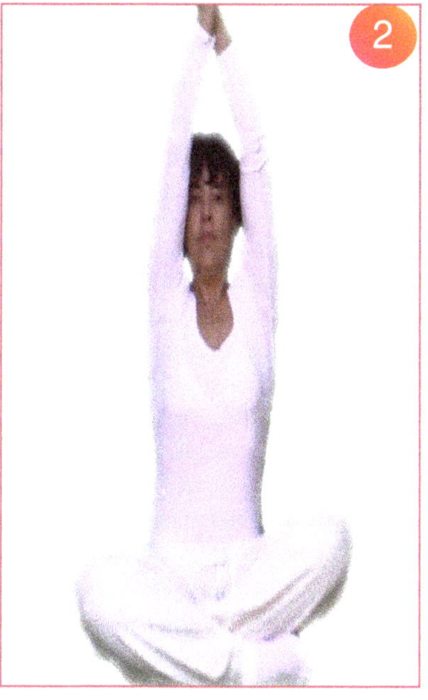

35. 9° EXERCISE FOR THE COLON:

PUMPING THE NAVEL

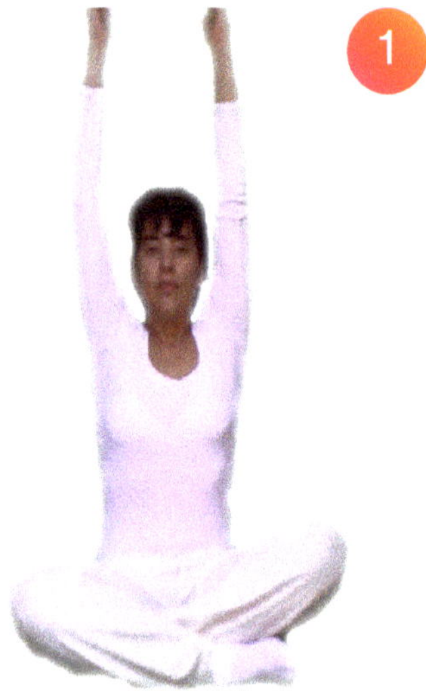

1) Sit in a comfortable position, inhale deeply and stretch your arms upward.

Exhale completely. Then inhale deeply and pump the navel for 6 seconds.

Repeat this exercise twice.

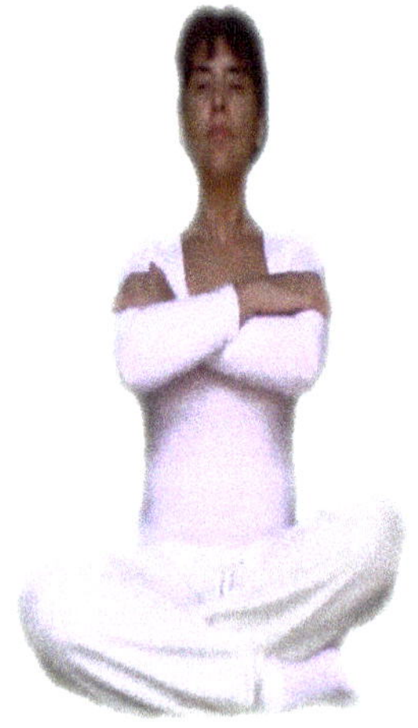

2) Now cross your arms in front of you so that each of your hands is on the opposite arm.

Inhale deeply and pump the navel at a slow pace (20 to 30 times).

Then exhale.

Inhale again and pump the navel again the same amount of times.
Perform this exercise for 3 minutes.

36. 10° EXERCISE FOR THE COLON: CHILD'S POSE

Remain in this position, the child's pose, for 5 minutes. Breathe slowly and deeply through your nose during the exercise.

Sit on your knees.

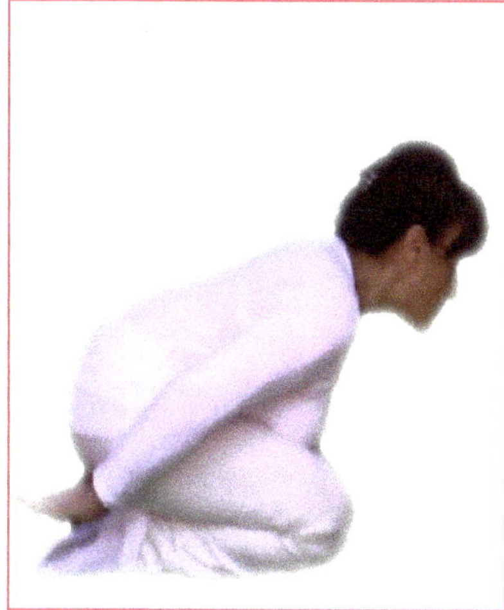

1) Exhale and let your back down while stretching it.

2) Stretch until your forehead touches the floor. Ensure that you're not lifting your buttocks from your ankles.

Shoulders should remain relaxed and your arms should be at your sides.

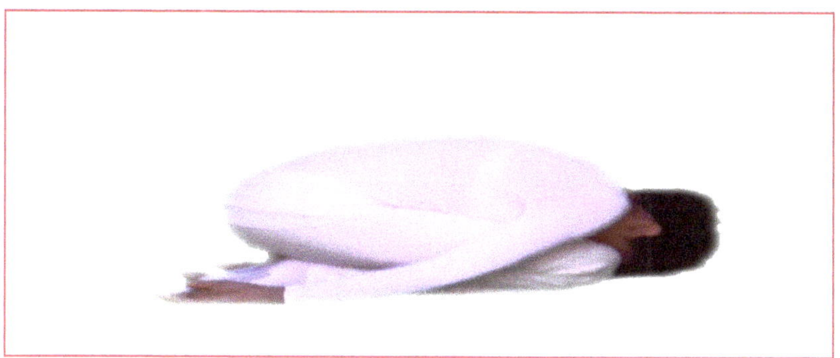

37. MEDITATION THAT HEALS NEUROSES AND ADDICTIONS

This healing meditation against neuroses and addictions must be done for 5-7 minutes. With practice, the time can be increased to 20 - 31 minutes. It is particularly effective against all types of addictions, because the pressure exerted by the action of inches and mandibles frees a certain rhythm in the brain.

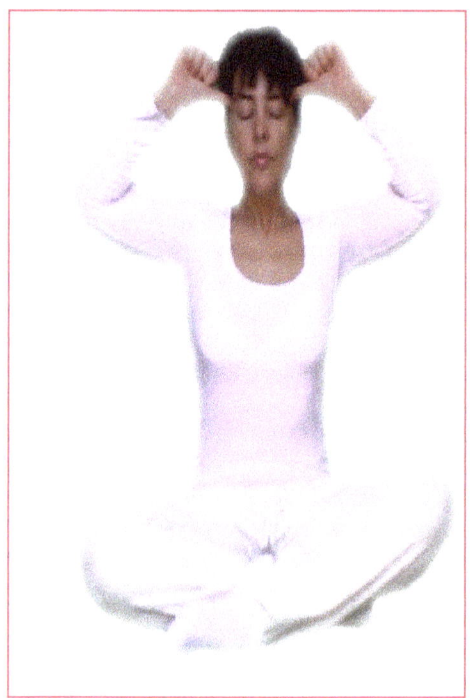

This rhythm activates the area directly at the base (stalk) of the pineal gland (epiphysis), facilitating the synchronization between the pineal and pituitary glands and correcting the problem of addictions.

Sit in a comfortable pose with the back straight. Make your hands into fists with your thumbs up. Place your thumbs on the cavity of your temples and apply firm pressure. With lips closed, tighten the muscles of the jaws alternating pressure on the molars. Feel the muscles move rhythmically under his fingertips.

Keep your eyes closed and concentrate on the third eye (the point between your eyebrows). Breathe deeply through your nose mentally coordinating your breath with the mantra SA TA NA MA during the inhalation and SA TA NA MA during the exhalation.

38. FIRST CHAKRA: VARIATION OF THE POSITION OF CROW

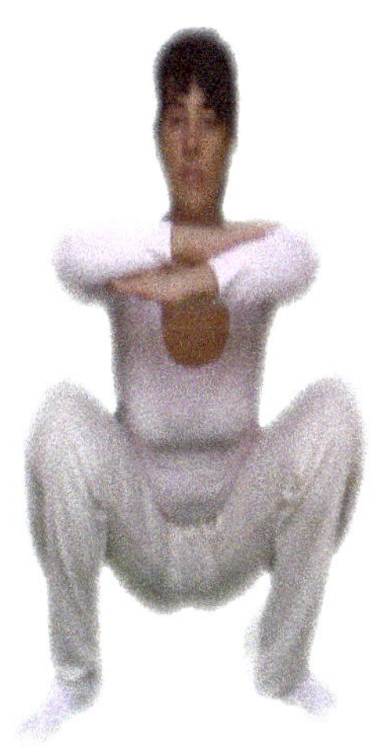

1) Squat on the floor and spread you legs so that your feet are about 40 cm (16 in) apart.
The soles of your feet should be on the ground and the points of your feet should be facing outwards. Your spine should be straight, your chin slightly raised and your arms in front of you and parallel to the ground.

2) Inhale as you stand up. Then exhale as you go back into a squatting position (always keeping your arms parallel to the ground). Continue this exercise for 3 minutes.

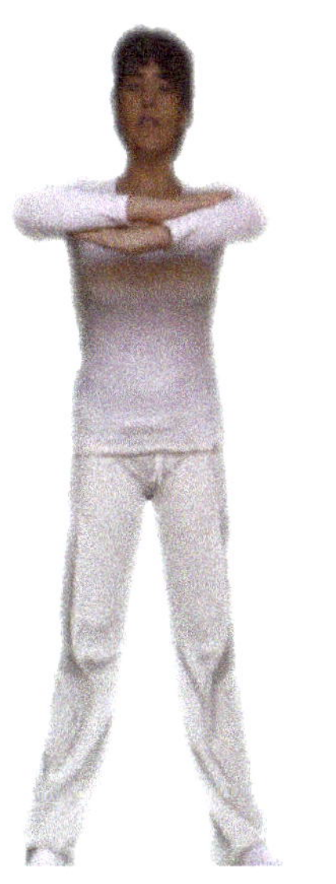

The Crow's position should only be done after you are already warmed up. The pose of the crow is a rather active position, it opens the base chakra, giving you a sense of security, ease, and grounding. It increases flexibility in the groin and hips, strengthens the gastrointestinal system, the knees and the ankles.

39. FIRST CHAKRA: STRETCHING FORWARD

This posture promotes the stretching of the sciatic nerve, which is important to increase physical energy.
Also it is used in the treatment of constipation, hemorrhoids and impotence, because it acts on energy elimination.
Do this exercise for 1 minute at each side.

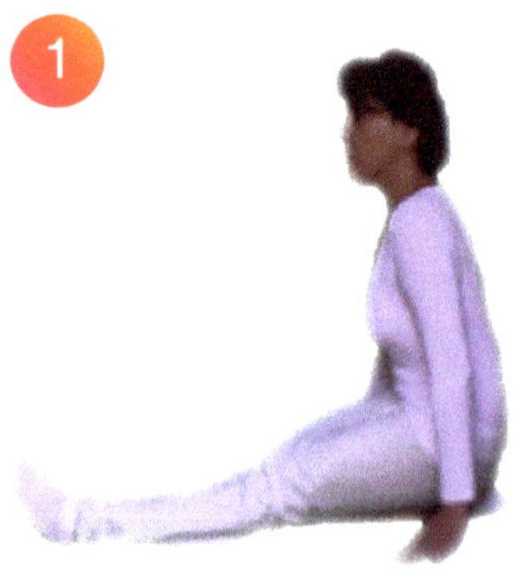

1) Sit with your legs stretched out in front of you. Bend your right knee and place the heel between the genitals and anus. This is a position that puts pressure on the CV1 point, corresponding to the sacral plexus and the base of the column.

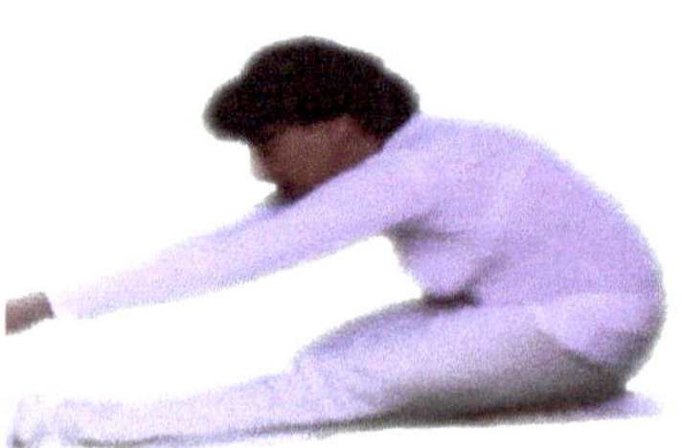

2) With your left leg stretched out, grab your shin or ankle as you inhale deeply.
Exhale as you bring your forehead towards your left knee. Do 1 minute on each side. Breathe slowly and deeply through your nose throughout this exercise.

40. FIRST CHAKRA: VARIATION OF THE POSITION OF THE CHAIR

The position of the chair has an effect on the kidneys, the upper part of the legs, the meridian of the large intestine, and the abdominal organs. Do this exercise for 1 and a half minutes to 3 minutes. As usual breathe slowly and deeply trough your nose.

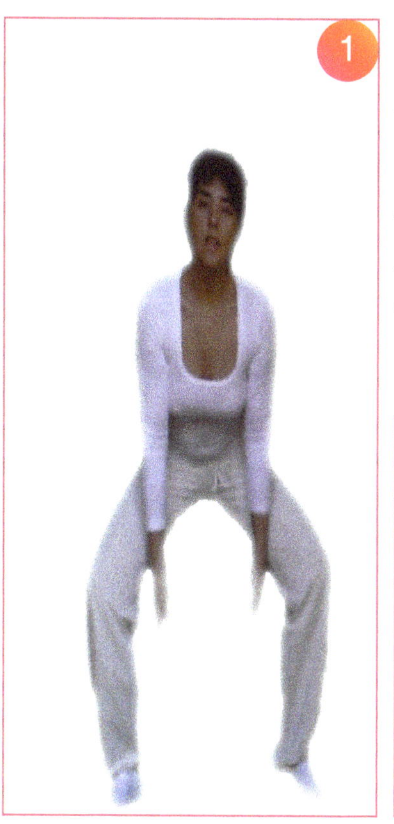

1) From a standing position, bend your back forwards until it is parallel with the ground. You can bend your legs a bit as well.

2) Now bring your arms through the inside of your legs, behind and around your calves and place your hands over your feet.

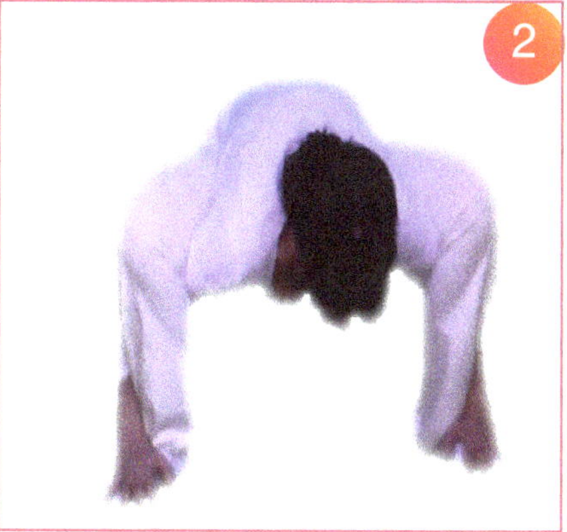

41. FIRST CHAKRA: VARIATION OF THE POSITION OF THE CAMEL

Time: 1 minute.

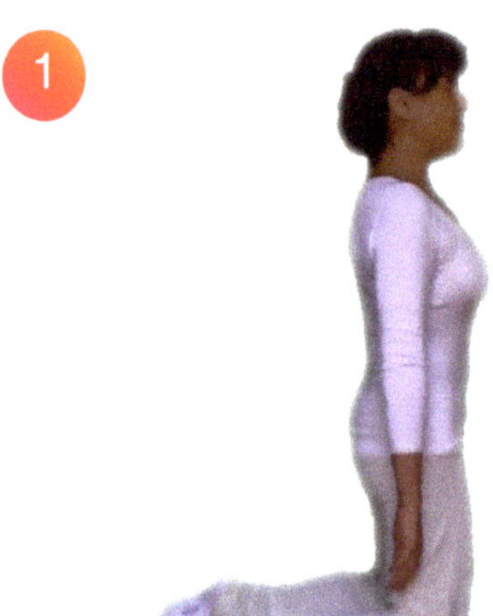

1) Sit on your heels, and have your knees shoulder-width apart.

2) Place your hands on your lower back and arch your back as much as possible.

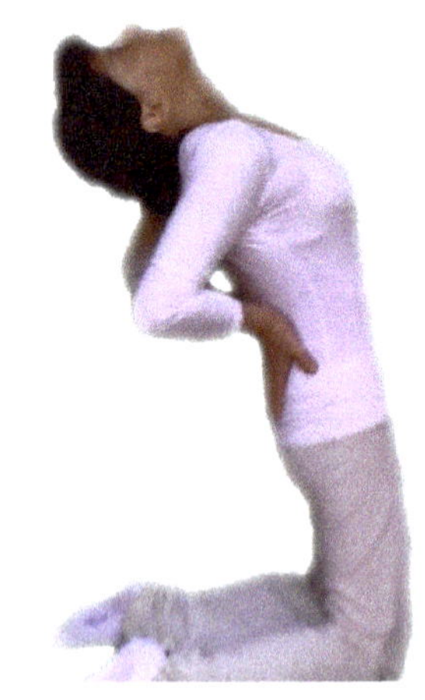

Your head should relax backwards as your hips push forward.
Breathe slowly and deeply through your nose.

42. FIRST CHAKRA: VARIATION OF THE POSITION OF THE COBRA

The position of the cobra is very useful to develop the torso and chest. It will also relieve tension on your neck and your back, as well as tighten your arms and buttocks.

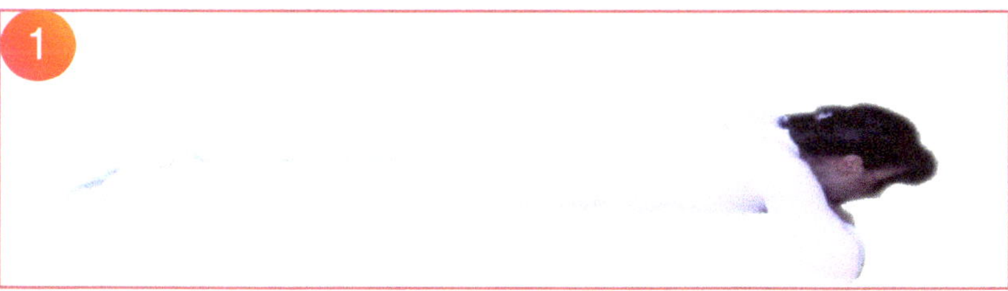

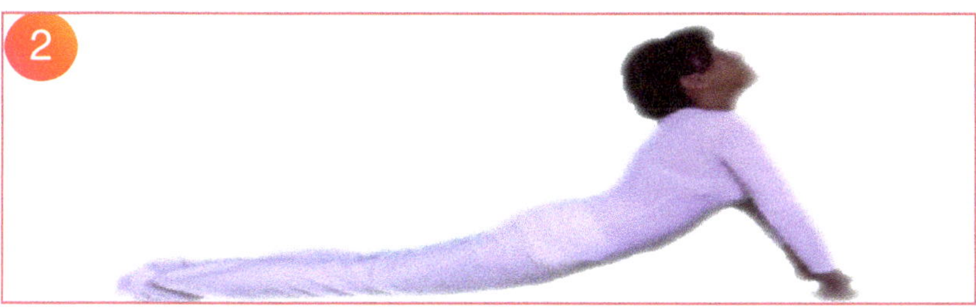

1) Lie on your abdomen. Bring your forehead to the ground. Put your hands under your shoulders; the tips of your fingers should be touching together.

2) Bend your head back. Then inhale as you lift your whole torso backwards with the help of your arms. Do not force this movement, simply go as far as you can.

Then lower your torso slowly as you exhale. Place your left cheek on the floor and relax your arms.

Repeat this exercise 2 more times.

43. FIRST CHAKRA: POSITION OF THE FROG

Perform this exercise for 5 minutes.

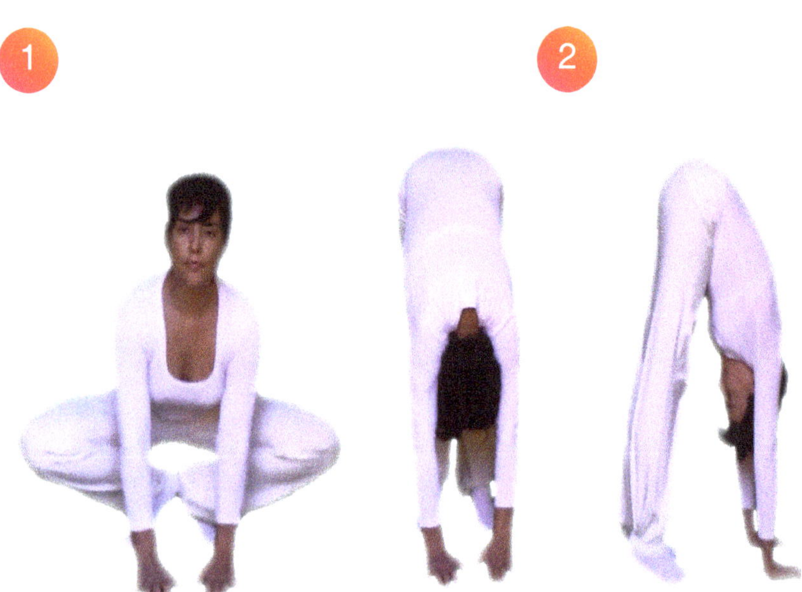

1) Squat on your toes (keep your heels touching). Your hands should also be placed on the floor in front of you.

2) As you inhale straighten your legs and lift your heels off the ground.

Then, as you exhale, return your legs to the initial squatting position, and return your spine to a straight position.

44. First Chakra: the drop

This exercise works on the GV1, an acupressure point located at the base of the spine; then it acts on the sacral plexus and promotes the development of the inner harmony, stability and safety.

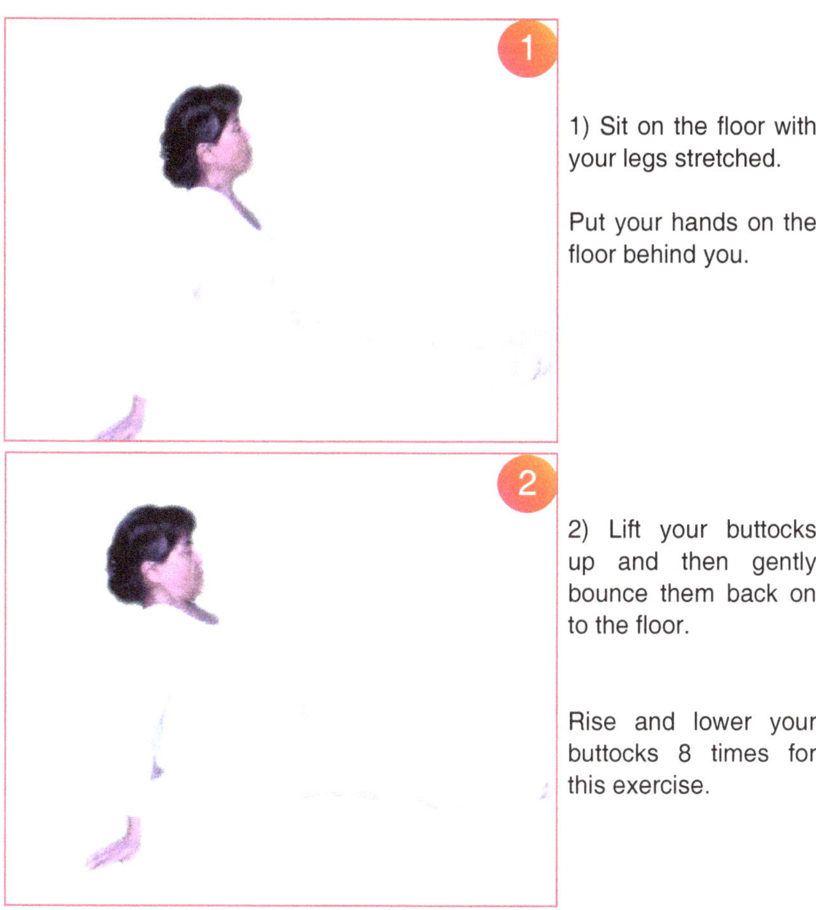

1

1) Sit on the floor with your legs stretched.

Put your hands on the floor behind you.

2

2) Lift your buttocks up and then gently bounce them back on to the floor.

Rise and lower your buttocks 8 times for this exercise.

45. FOURTH CHAKRA: BEAT OF WINGS

This exercise is very useful to fight a feeling of heaviness in the chest, and if you have difficulty breathing or to lower the blood pressure.
Perform this exercise for 3 minutes.

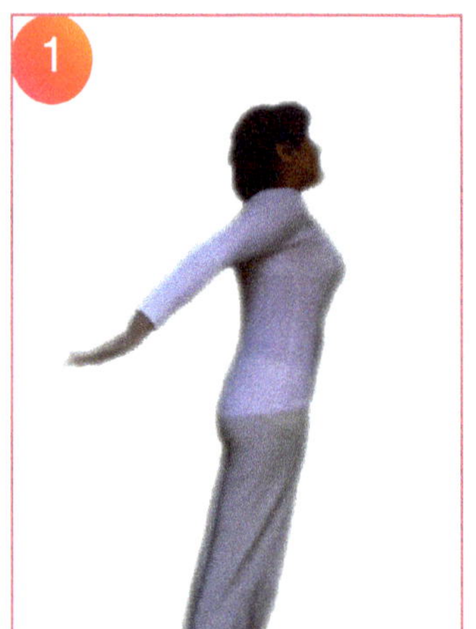

1) Standing up, bring your arms parallel to the ground, with your palms facing up.

As you inhale stretch your arms straight backwards (until you feel a bit of pressure on your shoulders and wrists) and then bring your chest up and forward.

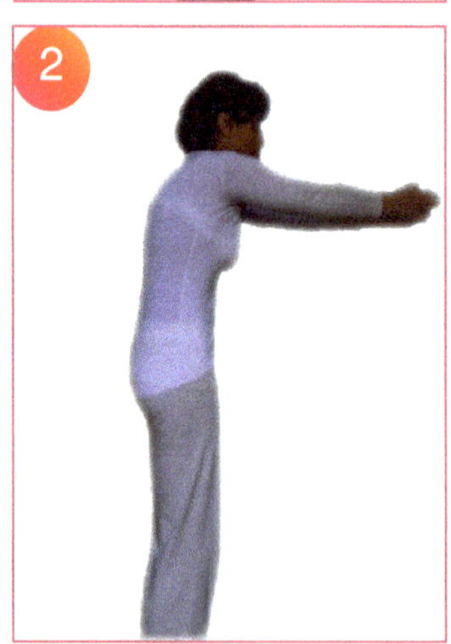

2) As you exhale bring your arms forward (while keeping them straight).

Place your hands together, palm to palm in front of you and arch your back forwards.

You want to be inhaling while your hands go backwards and exhaling when your hands go forwards.

46. FOURTH CHAKRA: HEARTBEAT

Meditate in the following position for 3 minutes. In this position you should be able to feel your heartbeat. This posture gives you a great sense of tranquillity and warmth because it connects together the starting and the ending points of the Heart Meridian.

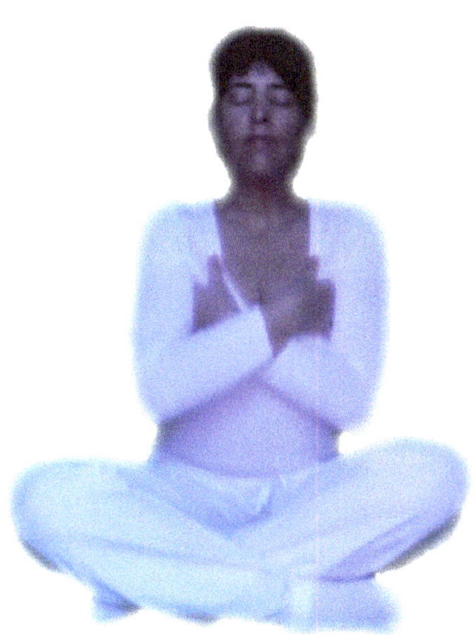

Sit in a comfortable pose with your back straight. Put your right hand under your left armpit and your left hand under your right armpit.

Close your eyes and concentrate on your heartbeat.

47. FOURTH CHAKRA: MEDITATION IN PRAYER POSE

Meditate in this position for 3 minutes.

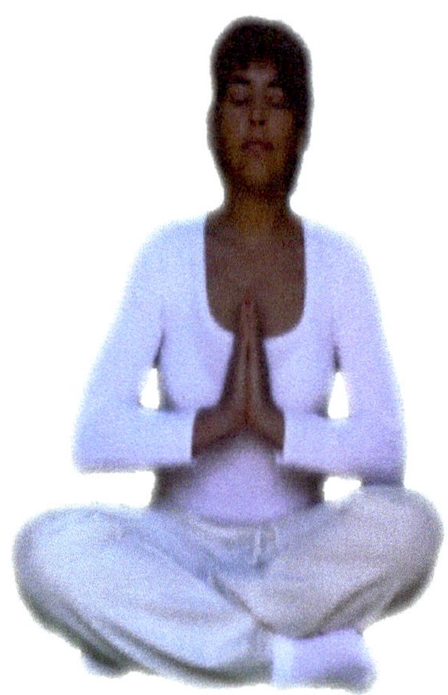

Sit in a comfortable pose. Keep your hands in prayer position at the center of your chest.

Perform 4 to 8 breathing: inhale through your nose for 4 seconds and then exhale through your nose for 8 seconds.

Either focus on the "third eye" point or the brow point (at the top of the nose where the eyebrows meet).

48. FOURTH CHAKRA: MEDITATION ON THE BEAT

This meditation requires some will power to perform consistently, but if done regularly it will clear your subconscious and any external behavior from disharmony and confusion. As written in the texts of kundalini yoga, this exercise is so powerful that if the worst criminal did it for 90 consecutive days for 2½ hours a day, he would abandon all aggressive behaviors.

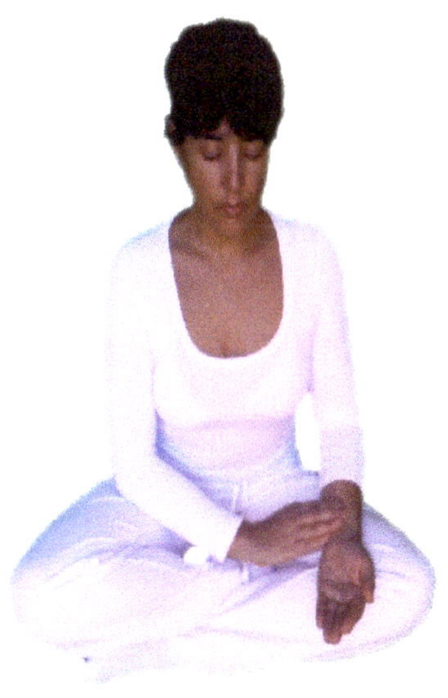

Sit in a comfortable position with your back straight.

Put your left arm on your left thigh with the palm facing up.

Place the four fingers of your right hand on the pulse of your left hand.

Feel your pulse on your left wrist.

To do this properly your pinky should be the one closest to the wrist.

Only your fingertips should be touching your arm.
Close your eyes and meditate while listening to your pulse. On each beat of the heart, mentally hear the sound "Sat Nam".

Your beats should do "japa" (repeat a mantra in meditation).
Don't do anything other than listening to your heartbeat.

49. FOURTH CHAKRA: TALK TO YOUR HEART

This meditation uses a sound to nourish the fourth chakra, the energy center of the heart.

Stay in this position for 3 minutes while listening to the vibrations that the sound 'Yahhmm' creates in your heart.

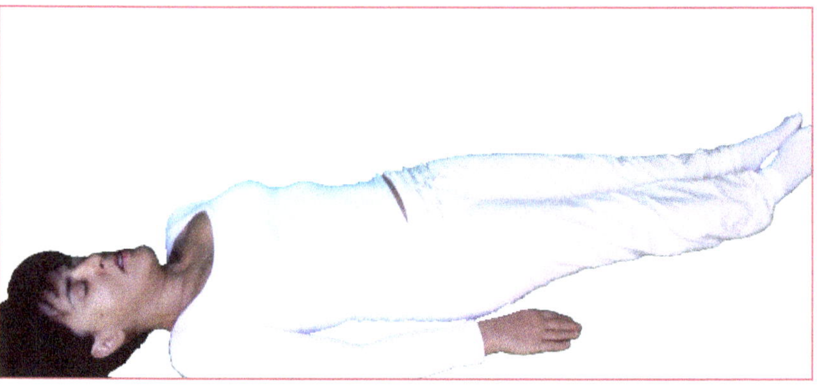

Stay in this position for 3 minutes while listening to the vibrations that the sound 'Yahhmm' creates in your heart.

Lie on your back.

Close your eyes and relax your body.

Inhale deeply and as you exhale chant the sound "Yahhmm".

50. AUTHOR'S NOTE

Yoga has been truly beneficial in my life because it helped me overcome some difficult times.

After my first book: "Bulimia - Come lo yoga mi ha aiutato", I decided to write this second book about yoga, where I have now shared my experiences.

The exercises on this book are a huge help for my students and I.

These exercises give us the gift of having balance in our lives even during situations which are not easy at all.

After my degree and journalistic work, I attended a school which allowed me to become a certified teacher of Kundalini Yoga (Certificate recognized internationally by IKYTA-KRI, USA and national by IKYTA Italy).

Then I took a diploma in sports, beauty, anti-stress, decontracting massage and I did a year of Shiatsu (Italian Academy Shiatsu-Do).

After these studies I decided to deepen my knowledge in several areas, such as: acu-yoga, yoga and meditation in the water, dance yoga, self shiatsu, the study of the meridians associated with traditional yoga and yoga for children.

It is always important for me to understand why each student wants to practice yoga.

My approach is to do a personalized study on their character, personality and individual needs, applying the findings in a program that can contain one or more disciplines, and that is specifically engendered to help that individual.

Dr. Roberta Grova
Web: robertagrova.com

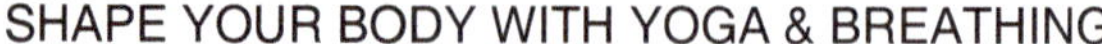

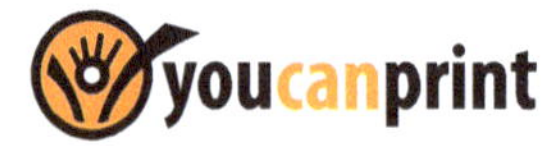

Finito di stampare nel mese di Maggio 2015
per conto di Youcanprint *Self-Publishing*